HEALTH & HUMAN NATURE

Health
&
Human
Nature

Paul Snyder

A FRANK E. TAYLOR BOOK

CHILTON BOOK COMPANY   RADNOR, PENNSYLVANIA

To the memory of my father
W. L. H. S.
1900–1940

47050 -2
R
733
S96
1980

6602224

CONTENTS

PREFACE

My professional interest is in the history of science and the philosophical underpinning of scientific thought. I became interested in holism initially because it seemed to me that this developing trend in medicine represented a clear-cut instance of a basic and important change in scientific concepts that could be studied as it happened rather than in retrospect. But it quickly became evident that the recent events in medical research are of more than philosophical interest, that the holistic approach to health and medicine had something to do with me personally, and that this way of thinking about human beings is relevant to the way I live and the decisions I make about my own health and well-being.

To study science is to study the activities of a community of tough-minded people who are constantly engaged in critical debate and experimentation, and who are careful about what they claim. Many of the serious scientists who comprise that community have changed their thinking about health and disease in recent years, and that change is reflected in their willingness to discuss and investigate questions that have not been asked before in the mainstream of Western medical science. But when medical people discuss their work, they tend to see the holistic movement as centering around their own research interests. They tend to lose sight of the fact that holism is as much a philosophical movement as a medical one, and as much a psychological movement as a biological one. All the human sciences have been affected by it, and this is only the beginning. To find the pattern, to fit specific research into a developing picture of human nature and the factors which influence our health, requires taking a philosophical step back from the scientific action and looking for the themes that tie together the new research in a variety of fields.

Holism, as a way of thinking about human beings, appears under several different labels in new approaches to medical practice: "Behavioral Medicine," "Humanistic Medicine," "Integral Medicine," and "Holistic (or Wholistic) Medicine." My aim in this book is to explain what holism is and why it has caught hold in the human sciences, and then to describe some significant recent developments in medical research and practice from a holistic point of view. Most of the medical information has been published before, in research reports or in isolated news stories. I have tried to tie those fragments together in such a way as to make sense of them, to describe the direction that professional health care seems to be taking, and to spell out the holistic basis for making sensible, responsible individual decisions about dealing with disease and about living a healthy life.

HEALTH & HUMAN NATURE

CHAPTER ONE

Holistic Medicine and Traditional Medicine

Shifting Points of View

The medical professions are in conflict now. They may well be in agony within the next decade. The argument is about a way of thinking called *holism*. It is reflected in some medical developments that are different from any we have seen before:

- Researchers at major medical schools are treating high blood pressure by teaching patients Oriental meditation techniques.
- Nutritionists warn that schizophrenia, anxiety neurosis, and suicidal depression may result from a poor diet.
- A psychiatrist claims that within five years we will be able both to predict and to detect cancer through personality tests.

- After generations of improvement in surgical techniques, health authorities now tell us to avoid surgery whenever possible.
- A famous surgeon finds that his patients heal faster if they believe that they will.
- A cancer researcher finds that some patients' tumors go away if they can imagine the right things and that aggressive people are more likely to recover from cancer than agreeable ones.
- Psychologists teach children with a blood disease how to hypnotize themselves in order to control internal bleeding.
- Medical people, philosophers, and psychologists claim that we can no longer make a distinction between the mind and the body.
- A vocal underground of nurses and an increasing number of physicians are talking about holistic medicine, about treating the whole person, not just the damaged parts. They say that your lifestyle—even if it is not obviously outrageous—is more likely to make you ill than any virus.

It's difficult to know just how seriously to take all the talk about holistic medicine and holistic approaches to health; difficult to understand the claim that the distinction between mind and body has broken down and that medicine and psychology must now deal with the "whole person," whatever that means. Does it make any sense? Can it possibly be a part of scientific medicine? Or is it just another fad?

Of course there are fads associated with the holistic movement in medicine and psychology. There are fads and fast-buck artists associated with anything that is new, especially when it has to do with health. But at its core, holism is not a fad. Take it seriously. It is a deep-seated and important change in the thinking behind scientific medicine. It isn't going to fade away like last year's fashions. It will affect the way you and I, our children and our grandchildren take care of ourselves, and it will affect the kinds of medical service that will be available in decades to come.

But what about right now? In almost every area of science that has to do with human well-being, there seem to be at least two reasonable and well-represented schools of thought. It isn't just a matter of the scientists denouncing dangerous and silly fads. Whether you are seeking expert advice about surgery, nutrition, vitamins, emotional problems, cancer, heart disease, or just a decent set of guidelines about the best way to take care of yourself, you find that the experts are deep in argument. Such arguments have happened before in science and they will happen again. Conflict and debate are a natural part of science. The dialogue and disagreement are vital to the process. The conservatism of the scientific community, its reluctance to change, saves us from the crackpots. The radicalism of the new proposals, the stinging denunciations of the established way of doing things, keep medical science growing and developing, and save it from stagnation.

It would be fascinating just to sit back and watch the argument, to observe the scientific debate in a detached way, except for one thing: the argument is about us, and about the best way for us to take care of ourselves. We can't just wait a few decades for the arguments to be settled; we have lives to live, and we need to make sound judgments now about the best way to live them.

You would think that after thousands of years of trying to understand nature we, or at least the scientists among us, would have an accurate description of the human system as it really is. But no accurate description of anything ever carries with it the guarantee that it is the *only* accurate description. There are always alternative ways to describe things and sort them out, and accuracy alone isn't generally what leads a scientist to prefer one way over another.

Scientific inquiry doesn't consist of simply watching the world, waiting for the truths of nature to reveal themselves. It consists of tackling the world with specific questions. We frame the questions, from whatever point of view seems reasonable to us. We determine what it is that we ask about. Observations, experiments, and tests must be devised to answer the questions we ask, the results must be interpreted, and arguments and criticisms must be brought to bear on those results to sort out the reasonable answers to our questions from the unreasonable ones. Science is a particular kind of human activity, a critical process by which we come to understand and manipulate natural forces. Changing circumstances, needs, and interests bring about corresponding changes in the point of view from which we approach nature—changes in the very concepts that we employ when we attempt to describe nature accurately. This means that scientists in every field ask different questions than their predecessors did. And different questions bring different answers.

Holism in medicine and psychology represents such a change in the character of scientific questions, and it is based upon a change in the conception of what it is that we study when we look at a person. The change shows up in at least three distinct principles that people in the human sciences have come to believe.

- First, a person is one thing, not two. The human mind and the human body can no longer be treated as two separate entities.
- Second, a person is not a set of distinct mechanisms, but a tightly organized biological unit.
- Finally, this biological unit must be understood in the setting in which its life takes place. It is dependent upon a set of ecological relationships with the rest of the world.

The Mechanistic Tradition

As reasonable as these three holistic principles may seem, they constitute a significant departure from the approach to health and medical research that has become established in Western countries over the past several hundred years. Because of the great successes of modern scientific medicine, many medical professionals are reluctant to embrace holistic principles. They believe that scientific medicine is a new thing in human history, that ignorance and superstition dominated medicine until very recently and are constantly threatening to take it over again. A recent editorial in the *New England Journal of Medicine* warns that the "worthwhile philosophy of holism" is likely to be abused by those who seek "quick solutions to all the ills of mankind through the abandonment of science and rationality in favor of mystical cults."[137] In response, others argue that some modes of treatment which are accepted without question today were considered "mystical" and highly suspicious by the scientific community of a hundred years ago.[85]

Some medical writers believe that scientific medicine, and perhaps all of science, is an invention of Western culture, and that it didn't begin at all until the past two or three hundred years. That is simply false. Science, in the clearest sense, consists of the systematic development of group solutions to common problems. Criticism, dialogue, debate, disagreement, testing and experimentation are what it takes to hone and refine the ideas of individuals and integrate them into a systematic body of useful knowledge. For as long as people have been living in communities, they have been carrying out scientific activity. The theories of our sciences represent, at any given time and place, the best collective understanding that we have of the world, of *how* to direct natural forces to our advantage, how to predict what will happen if we do specific things, and how to explain what has happened in the past so that we can plan our future activities.

From the very beginning, our understanding of ourselves has always been an integral part of our understanding of nature in general. Of course there has always been a body of unscientific lore that is best identified as "folk medicine." But for at least 2500 years there has also been a solid tradition of medicine that was linked to the rest of science, and that changed and developed as the rest of science did. As techniques and conceptions changed, many beliefs that began in the realm of folk medicine were brought into the mainstream of established and tested knowledge, and many others that did not stand up to criticism and testing were dropped.

We tend to concentrate on the failures of past science, on the quaint ideas that were introduced to explain how and why the world worked. We often forget the successes, developed within an understanding of nature that was different from that of contemporary science. They made possible developments in navigation, agriculture, engineering, and mechanics, and in health and medicine as well. They laid the foundation of modern civilization and they shaped our way of thinking.

For almost two thousand years, from the time of Aristotle to the time of Rene Descartes and Isaac Newton, Western thought conceived nature as a great organism, and human beings were understood to be the central part of that organism. The scientific questions had to do with the order, function, and purpose of specific things in the overall scheme of nature. Inanimate objects like rocks and bits of metal were understood to be at some pre-organic stage of development. The point of reference was organic life, and the scientific questions were the same for the organs of the human body, for the stones and the marine life along the Mediterranean coast, and for the stars in the night sky: where does this item fit in the scheme of living things? What is its nature, its function? What kind of balance does it strike with the other items around it? How is that balance preserved, and how does it change? Such questions dominated scientific inquiry in North Africa, Europe and the Middle East.

In medicine as well as in physics, botany, astronomy, and chemistry, the questions were often answered. Specific treatments for specific illnesses were developed, systematized, and catalogued by the physician Galen in the second century, along with tested techniques for dealing with wounds and injuries. A long line of successors extended and amplified Galen's work, right up to the seventeenth century.

Then, in a period much like the present, science shifted ground. Between 1500 and 1700 there was a sharp change in the character of scientific questions. In all the sciences, there was as much turmoil and change in that period as there has been in the twentieth century. Technical developments came rapidly. As life became more complicated and trade and exploration increased, people needed to know *how* things worked rather than why. The scientific questions moved, a notch at a time, from questions of order and function to questions of mechanics and physical relationships. In every area of science, the question became *How do things work?* By 1650, the tone was set that was to dominate Western science right up to the beginning of our own century: the world was to be studied as a great mechanism. Not just the solar system, not just the motions of projectiles and falling bodies, but everything, including plants, animals, and the human system, now had to be understood in mechanical terms. The heart came to be understood as part of a hydraulic system, the lungs as an air pump. The breath of life, the *pneuma* that was believed to separate living things from dead things, came to be understood as a simple atmospheric gas, composed of mechanically interacting particles of matter. Once Isaac Newton had nailed down the growing conception of nature in one neat, compact set of physical laws, it became an article of faith that there was a mechanism behind every natural process.

The constant search for the mechanism within the mechanism, for the invisible particles whose mechanical action produced the visible characteristics of living things, led to the discovery of the cell structure of the human body, and this in turn led to the discovery of the tiny organisms which attacked the cells and damaged or destroyed them. One after another, the infectious diseases that could not have been understood and treated by asking about the function and balance of the human body yielded to the mechanical line of attack. The human system, viewed in isolation from the world around it, was analyzed into more and more minute mechanisms. It was understood to be a machine like any other machine; perhaps a little more complicated, but still a machine.

In this past century, science in general has outgrown mechanism. Energy—heat, light, electricity, magnetism and radio-activity—simply cannot be understood in purely mechanical terms. Despite the many developments for harnessing energy that made the machine age possible, the mechanical analysis ultimately reached its limits. Although most natural systems can be treated as machines, the particles which constitute matter are not physical objects of any sort that a Newtonian could recognize, and they do not relate to each other in a mechanical way.

Scientific thinking is not necessarily mechanistic thinking anymore. To tackle a question scientifically is to tackle it critically and responsibly, to put our ideas forward bravely and subject them to the testing and criticism that are only available where there is a scientific community. And scientific thinking isn't infallible. It doesn't represent eternal truth. There is no reason to believe that the most recent changes in scientific thought will be the last ones. Nevertheless, we make plans, decide matters of public policy, and even stake our lives on particular courses of action based upon the current scientific conceptions of the world. We are able to do so because any insight that we turn up concerning the world and our place in it has to be subjected to criticism and testing by a stubborn and tough-minded scientific community before it is incorporated into the body of information we call scientific knowledge.

Mechanism was the style of the Western scientific community for almost 300 years. By understanding nature as a great machine, we were able to solve scientific problems that could not be tackled with the earlier organic conception of nature. And because mechanism generated problems of its own, every one of the natural sciences has turned away from it in this century.

Still, don't give too much attention to those who glibly denounce the mechanistic approach to science and medicine. Most of us wouldn't be alive and coping without the fruits of precisely the kind of science that brought about improvements in sanitation and nutrition, and the fruits of the kind of medicine that went on to identify the agencies that cause specific diseases and to develop means for the prevention and cure of those diseases.[111] The triumph of the mechanistic tradition of medicine lay in the development of surgical procedures for repairing damage, for removing diseased tissue, and for overcoming infection. Modern chemical and drug therapies are a direct outgrowth of the intense analytic concentration on cell structures and the organisms that can attack them. It would be absurd to exclude such items from the physician's repertoire, even though the hope of holistic medicine is eventually to develop a clear enough understanding of our own biological nature that we can safeguard against disease and deal with it effectively without such drastic intervention. But that time has not yet come, and we cannot abandon orthodox medical procedures that have proven effective, even if they are grounded in a mechanistic view of human beings that we no longer subscribe to. That would be like discarding the electric light because we understand electricity in a different way than Edison did. To acknowledge a change in medical and scientific thinking, we do not have to deny the value of everything that has gone before. We have to absorb it into the new scheme of things.

It's not that Newtonian science was wrong; it wasn't. Newton developed a perfect physics for dealing with mechanical systems. But we know now that not all systems are mechanical. There is another physics beyond mechanistic physics. We can't look at the universe as a great machine anymore.

And we can't look at ourselves that way, either. There is now another medicine beyond mechanistic medicine. It is called holistic medicine.

Minds, Bodies, and Persons

When you talk about yourself, what are you talking about? A mind? A body? Both? Or something quite different? How you answer those questions is going to affect what you believe about yourself, and what you are willing to say about mankind in general. More important, the way medical and psychological researchers answer those questions is going to affect the kind of research that is done and the kind of information and guidance that is available to us about how to take care of ourselves.

Three hundred years ago, when Descartes attempted to sort out theological issues from scientific ones, he argued that the human soul was something separate from the mechanism of the body, that is was not subject to mechanical laws, and that science could not study it. The task of any proper scientist was to work out the mechanical principles by which God had created the physical world. It didn't even make sense to ask about connections between psychological events and bodily processes.

The biggest problem with Descartes' manifesto for science isn't that he made too sharp a distinction between soul and body, but that he made no distinction at all between soul and mind. Whatever religious beliefs one might hold about immortal souls, it isn't the soul that is impaired when a person receives a brain-damaging injury, and it isn't the soul that gets drunk or tranquilized or high on marijuana. It isn't the soul that perceives a particular situation as threatening and initiates the physiological changes that enable us to cope with the threat, and it isn't the soul that gets tense enough to cause ulcers. None of these matters have anything to do with souls or immortality; they have to do with the mundane, day-to-day business of living a life.

In time, what Descartes began as an attempt to exempt the immortal soul from scientific scrutiny became a fragmentation of the mortal human self into two separate and distinct things, a mind and a body. While some scientists tried to explain all mental events as physical processes—simply the action of a much more complicated machine than even Descartes could have imagined—most thought that the physical machine could be isolated, and that it was the only proper object of scientific study.

One major recent attempt to come to grips with human activity—as distinct from the supposed mechanism itself—is the movement in psychology known as *behaviorism*. Behaviorism watches the machine do things; it studies human beings as behaving bodies, and seeks to establish the ways in which the human machine tends to respond to particular stimuli. In its more radical forms, it attempts to do away with all mentalistic concepts and speak only of overt behavior and the publicly observable causes of that behavior.

But as the philosopher Herbert Feigl has observed, the causal factors which determine human behavior include such activities as "planning, deliberation, preference, choice, volition, pleasure, pain, displeasure, love, hatred, attention, vigilance, enthusiasm, grief, indignation, expectations, remembrance, hopes, wishes, and so on."[55] All of these are inaccessible to a purely behavioristic psychology.

Behaviorism in psychology is like Newtonian mechanism in

physics. It isn't that there is no value to it, not that it is dead wrong as far as it goes, but rather that there has to be another psychology beyond it. There are legitimate questions that need to be answered about the connections between the human characteristics on that long list of Herbert Feigl's and the overall health and well-being of the human beings who have those characteristics. Such questions can't be approached from a behavioristic point of view, because they can't even be asked; the characteristics cannot be dealt with at all. You just can't study a whole human being by looking only at overt behavior.

What has only recently begun to catch on is a serious attempt to abandon the mind-body distinction altogether. You don't *disprove* a distinction in science the way you disprove a hypothesis. You simply stop making the distinction when it ceases to be appropriate. The attempt began in earnest about thirty-five years ago with the rise of *psychosomatic* medicine. The premise of the psychosomatic approach was that the mind and the body could and did influence each other, contrary to what Descartes and his successors had thought. All of us now realize what isolated individuals suspected a long time ago: such diseases as asthma, peptic ulcers, colitis, rheumatoid arthritis, high blood pressure, and diseases of the heart and circulatory system are aggravated by anxiety and depression, and are very likely brought about by them. The psychosomatic approach made it possible to submit such a claim to systematic criticism and testing in clinical situations.

But the psychosomatic approach to disease didn't go far enough. It still had us implicitly trying to make a connection between two things—a body on the one side and a mind on the other—rather than two characteristics of the same thing: a person's emotional states and habits, and that same person's state of health.

From the psychosomatic beginnings, the shift to holism

in the mainstream medical literature has been steadily increasing. In 1974, Nobel laureate Nikolaas Tinbergen told the scientific community that "too rigid a distinction between body and mind is of only limited use to medical science, and in fact can be a hindrance to its advance."[172] Holism deals with a person as a functioning unit. If it is useful, this unit can be viewed from different angles, including a mental angle and a physical one. But these are still views of one entity: a person.

The term "person" was brought into the literature of philosophical psychology by Peter F. Strawson back in the 1950s.[106] Strawson attempted to spell out the logical and philosophical arguments in favor of a concept of the person as a single entity to which one can ascribe both states of consciousness and bodily characteristics. He argued compellingly that these two sets of characteristics need not be understood as functions of two separate entities. This argument is still developing on the borderline between the human sciences and philosophy. What is at issue are not the facts about human beings, but rather the concepts that we apply when we try to describe those facts in a systematic way.

More recently, American philosopher Joseph Margolis has tried to spell out the implications for psychology of the essentially holistic conception of a person.[106] Any study of the sensations, beliefs, perceptions and deliberate actions of human beings is going to be strongly influenced by the conceptual base on which that study is constructed, and by the questions it makes sense to ask about people when those concepts are applied to real situations. There are things characteristic of a person that can't properly be attributed either to a mind or to a physical mechanism. Both individually and collectively, we understand and follow rules, use language, make decisions about how to act, act sometimes on pure gut feelings or by enculturated habit, wonder, worry, and argue about what we should do, make judgments about ourselves and about each other, make choices, and take responsibility, get depressed or anxious, and influence each other's beliefs, feelings, and actions. Any of the "social" or "human" sciences must be able to make sense of these activities of whole people. And it is clear that medicine must make sense of them too.

From now on, I want to speak only of persons and their activities, rather than trying to speak about what the mind does or what the body does. Some activities, like pumping hormones, secreting bile, generating white blood cells, digesting food, and growing toenails, are things that a person ordinarily does unconsciously and involuntarily. Others, like holding the breath, raising an arm, working out a math problem, or deciding what to have for dinner, are things that a person ordinarily does consciously and deliberately.

What we take to be good for ourselves, what we think we can do, and what we are therefore willing to be held responsible for, depend on what we think we are. Looking at ourselves as persons has advantages. It gives us a way to make sense of many new medical developments, and provides a basis for making some decisions. It even makes us look at processes like digesting food or generating blood cells a little differently. Processes are impersonal and automatic; you can't ask who is responsible for them. But let's speak of them as activities, something you do. *You* digest your food, and in doing so you're involved in some activities over which you have conscious control, like chewing and swallowing. You generate red blood cells. And even though this activity isn't something that you can directly decide to do or not to do, some of the things you *can* decide about—eating or avoiding some foods, getting rest and exercise, and so on—will have an effect on the way you generate red blood cells.

A mind can have a grudge, and a body can have a broken rib. A person, something like you and me, can have both, and might have to deal with both over the course of a lifetime.

A person is also a cultural entity. We are the beings who think and use language. Beyond that, each of us has a *way* of thinking and talking about ourselves and our experiences that can be understood only by seeing the person within an overall cultural setting. Our natural environments include other persons and institutions, as well as sources of nourishment, air, and water, learned habits of activity and rest—the whole complicated set of relationships and interactions that go into living a life.

A major complaint against modern Western medicine is that it isolates the individual patient from the natural setting of life, that it removes a person from the setting in which disease developed, treats and repairs the organic damage to whatever extent it can, and pays no attention to the overall matrix of personal habit or the complex relationships between the person and the world that brought about the disease in the first place. At its worst, this approach to disease yields what critics call "symptom medicine"—the overall disorder is not treated, but only the symptoms or the damage that result from the disorder. It seems futile to use medication to lower a person's blood pressure if you don't at the same time tackle the characteristics of the person's life that raised the blood pressure in the first place.

Assembling the Holistic Picture

A conference sponsored in 1974 by the Rockefeller Foundation, Blue Cross, and the Health Policy Program of the University of California came up with four specific commitments that are involved in the shift to a holistic approach to human health.[33]

First is the matter of understanding that disease involves the total person. It is people who get sick, not organs and cells. Interventions in the course of disease must be made simultaneously from a number of angles, including those that are traditionally identified as emotional, cognitive, and physical. How you feel, what you believe about yourself, *and* what your lab tests show are all relevant to your state of sickness or health.

Second, understanding a person's state of health means understanding the immediate circumstances of the person's life—the substances used and handled at work, the foods available and the actual quality of nourishment, the habits of rest, the pressures of day-to-day living and the means available for relieving those pressures, and the presence and absence of all sorts of pollutants.

Third, what about the social and cultural environment? What kind of setting do we live in? As will become clear in the following chapters, the web of relationships, expectations, emotional patterns, and sheer habits of living that together constitute the picture of each human life are much more relevant to the state of our health than has previously been supposed.

Finally, and perhaps most important of all, is the matter of each individual assuming responsibility for the state of his own health. There are circumstances in every life that are beyond individual control, including, of course, pollution and the presence of carcinogens, as well as the economic and political facts which affect each of us. But how we cope with those circumstances in our individual lives on a day-to-day basis is up to us. The overall quality of life is up to us, individually, to maintain. Beyond that, there are specific and surprising connections between a person's *attitude* of self-determination and the way that person reacts to disturbing elements in the environment. The likelihood of your contracting disease, and the likelihood of your recovering from diseases you do contract, are strongly influenced by the extent to which you can take charge of your own habits, feelings, and circumstances.

The very term *patient* has its roots in the notion that we are passive to the ministrations of medical professionals when it comes to combatting disease. We have come to view disease as something that happens to us, and we tend to seek someone to "fix" what's wrong with us. In a holistic picture, the patient must become the *agent,* the active element in maintaining good health and overcoming disease. To do this, we need information. We must be informed about what does and what does not contribute to overall health, and what constitutes a constructive approach to overcoming disease. We must be able to sort out reliable information from fads and inflated or over-simplified claims. We must make sound judgments and assume responsibility for our own welfare. We need to make responsible decisions about when it is appropriate to seek professional medical intervention, and we need to know when and how to intervene in the course of our own lives and change our habits or circumstances.

The holistic conception of the person has distinct implications for the medical professions, although I think it is too early to claim that a New Medicine has taken over in Western culture. But there are startling new questions being asked and answered by medical researchers, questions that could not have been approached with the earlier mechanistic view of human beings. And as a result, there are new questions that all of us have to ask and answer for ourselves.

CHAPTER TWO

Our Biological Heritage

The Nature of the Beast

We like to think that human beings can shape and control the world. Since our ancestors first began to develop systematic agriculture about 10,000 years ago, we have built civilizations based on our increasing ability to understand natural forces and direct them to our advantage. This same ability has transformed the setting in which we live our lives into a world that our ancestors would not recognize.

At the same time, but at a much slower rate, the world shapes and controls us. Over millions of years the facts of life on this planet shaped our ancestors by the process of natural selection. But our activities and behavior, both individually and as a species, have changed at a much more rapid rate than our genetic makeup alone has. Over the centuries, we have selected techniques for living that have altered the quality of human life much more drastically than natural selection could possibly have altered us over the same period of time.

We are very much like those prehistoric farmers. Our natural abilities and needs are essentially the same as theirs. Like them, we are biologically equipped to be excellent hunters and gatherers of food. Our natural ways of marshaling our energies to deal with emergency, and the complex physiological responses that prepare us for specific kinds of activity and awareness, are precisely suited to that kind of life. But we simply do not know how well we are now suited biologically and behaviorally to the world our species has made so rapidly; the human sciences are just beginning to study the long-term consequences of the changes in diet, in daily activity, in the substances we use and handle daily, in the air we breathe and the water we drink, in our human relationships, in the ways we relieve tension, and in the emotional habits that constitute our personal adaptations to the world.

We need to develop a better understanding of our biological needs. In a very short period of evolutionary time, we have changed our environment, and we have changed the *way* we live in our environment to the extent that our own biological adaptation—our own nature—may be at odds with the world we have created. We need to get back in touch with nature, and by this I don't mean that we should return to the lifestyle of 9000 B.C. What we must do is develop a better sense of our own genetic adaptation, our capabilities for taking care of ourselves, and the limitations of what we can tolerate, and make those capabilities and limitations work for us, instead of against us.

Except for identical twins, no two people are genetically alike.[145] But despite the differences among us in minor structural elements, and despite the great genetic diversity within the human species, we are all the same *kind* of being, and we all face the same kind of problem in adjusting to the environment that we and our ancestors have created.

Our individual nutritional needs may be quite different, for example, but we can speak sensibly of the *range* of our individual requirements for specific vitamins, proteins, and other substances.[182] Our abilities are similar too, but they differ in relatively minor ways from one individual to another. Some people have the ability to do math problems in their heads; others can visualize whether the dining-room table will fit over in the far corner and still leave space for people to pass by on the way to the kitchen. Some of us can do neither very well. The same degree of variation occurs in our individual abilities to resist disease and to recover from it.

Beyond the genetic differences, each of us has learned to deal with day-to-day problems in individual ways, and this is reflected in the overall state of our health and in the way we respond to stress and disease.

Natural Remission and Other Non-Explanations

Some people never seem to be ill at all. Others become ill but recover quickly. Still others contract serious diseases that resist all medical treatment and then suddenly become well again in what their physicians call "natural" or "spontaneous" remission of symptoms. What this means, of course, is that the physician doesn't know why the patient recovered. Many such recoveries can be understood as the result of the natural workings of a person's resistance to disease. Lewis Thomas, commenting on the fact that physicians and their families tend to make less use of modern medical technology and surgery than most of the population does, notes: "The great secret, known to internists and learned in marriage by internists' wives, but still hidden from the general public, is that most things get better by themselves. Most things, in fact, are better by morning."[170]

When a person recovers from a serious, well-documented disease without medical treatment, or experiences a sudden and dramatic recovery after failing to respond to treatment for a long time, we ask why. Why did this person recover, and why doesn't everyone recover? Careful, serious studies of such matters are rare in medical literature. Many medical researchers doubt that such remission of verified symptoms *can* take place without specific therapy. They tend to doubt the original diagnosis or they attribute the symptoms to hysteria, self-hypnosis, or self-delusion. The scientific community dislikes open questions, and it therefore tends to doubt the existence of what it cannot explain. Those researchers who do speak of "spontaneous remissions" of disease, or who dismiss the remission of symptoms as "just hypnosis" or "all in the mind," are avoiding an important question. To label a person's disease psychosomatic or psychogenic, for example, shouldn't end the discussion of that disease, especially when clinically demonstrable symptoms are present.

In 1966 two separate studies were published about spontaneous recovery from cancer.[21,52] One study concluded that in the modern environment people are exposed to so many carcinogens that it is reasonable to suppose that everyone in his lifetime must develop one or more clusters of abnormal, cancerous cells, as well as such infections as tuberculosis. But this is no way to *end* such a study. We want to know what holds these diseases in check, what keeps them from spreading in most people, what enables most of us to destroy abnormal cells and infections. "When the clinician and experimentalist concentrate on immunity rather than on mortality . . . we may begin to think of the prevention, the control and the cure of cancer."[21]

The Immune System

Our primary natural means of self-defense against disease is a complex group of unconscious activities that are generally grouped together as the immune response. Its function is to maintain the integrity of the human system, to protect healthy cells and to destroy and remove foreign matter, viruses, bacteria, and unhealthy or abnormal cells. The business end of the immune system consists of mobile units of *immunocompetent* cells, cells that attack, destroy, and remove bits of matter that threaten the system. These mobile units are primarily *leukocytes,* or white blood cells, some of which can engulf and digest foreign or undesirable matter. Of these, *B cells* originate in bone marrow and *T cells* originate in the thymus gland.

Leukocytes are the first line of defense. They circulate through the bloodstream and are mobilized to specific trouble sites by the action of the hypothalamus region of the brain, an area under the cerebrum. Some of the cells are "imprinted" with the physical shape of specific organisms that they specialize in attacking. This imprinting is essentially what is involved in vaccination against a disease. Others are nonspecific and once they are activated, they will attack a variety of undesirable objects in the body. The cells are attracted to the site by the action of chemical signals released from tissues invaded by a pathogen (disease-causing substance).

If the pathogen is a bacterial colony, a substance in the blood called *opsonin* prepares and marks the bacteria for destruction. The bacteria are coated with antibodies and set up for the kill. The white blood cells—*phagocytes* or *macrophages*—recognize the alien cells by means of these chemical cues and attach themselves to them. Then they go on to kill the bacteria and digest them. (Here is one of those many stages in the physiology of human life where the textbooks all say "the complex biology of the process is not completely known," or "the mechanism is not well understood.") The cells then carry off the debris through the bloodstream, eventually to be eliminated from the body altogether.

The immune response is one way a person adapts to changes or threats in the daily course of events. The adaptation is neither deliberate nor conscious. If you have a splinter, you adapt to it by isolating it. Thousands of white blood cells, part of what we identify as pus, devour the bacteria that were carried in with the splinter. An abscess forms, gradually working the splinter and the fluids toward the surface of the skin. Eventually, in most cases, the abscess ruptures and discharges both the pus and the splinter. The whole process, uncomfortable though it might be, constitutes an unconscious adaptation to the invasion by the splinter. It is effective most of the time, and it is a matter of predictable routine in the involuntary housekeeping activities that we carry on constantly.

This complicated activity, which involves recognizing alien substances, weakening and labeling them for the kill, engulfing, digesting, and eventually disposing of them, is constantly going on. How well the immune system works against its marked enemies will of course determine the course of disease: whether there are no symptoms or many symptoms, whether complications are added to the effects of the pathogen itself by the extreme efforts of the immune system to deal with it, whether there is a chronic, recurring set of symptoms, speedy recovery, or, if it all fails, death.

The immune system can make mistakes, however. No biological activity is exempt from error. In some cases the immune system fails to recognize and attack the defective cells that constitute cancerous growths. In other cases the activity of the immune response is misdirected so that the T and B cells attack healthy tissue instead of disease organisms, resulting in what is known as auto-immune disease. In rheumatic fever, for example, the antibodies attack cells of the heart and the joints, apparently mistaking them for streptococcus organisms. Hay fever, some forms of anemia, lupus, and possibly multiple sclerosis and rheumatoid arthritis are all suspected to be auto-immune diseases.[65] The continuing research into immunity seeks to explain how the response succeeds in defending us against disease, why it sometimes fails, and why it sometimes actually turns against us.

Stress and Adaptation

More than any other species, we human beings are able to anticipate situations before they occur and prepare ourselves to deal with them. We aren't the only species that stores food for the winter, but we are the only species that can argue about *how* to store food for the winter in anticipation of the need to do so.

Moreover, each of us individually anticipates situations before they occur, and, like other animals, we react in predictable ways to situations that might pose a threat to our well-being. Threatening situations trigger an inborn and natural "fight-or-flight" response which is as much a part of our biological heritage as the immune response. And we share it with many other species. The cat with arched back and hair standing on end and the dog snarling at an unidentified movement are behaving in ways that are closely related to our own reaction to stressful situations. Blood pressure rises, breathing and heart rate increase, we "pump adrenalin," metabolism changes, and most of the digestive process comes to a halt as blood is directed to the muscles.

The successful use of all this preparation once determined the difference between life and death. It occurs to one degree or another whenever we prepare ourselves to deal with a challenge, whether or not the perceived challenge constitutes a real physical danger. We still get ourselves geared up in ways that are appropriate to fighting a saber-toothed tiger, when what we have to deal with is the plumber or the landlord. This is a sure way to generate stress, and this very protective stress leads to many of the diseases of civilized man. Only very recently has medicine developed any real understanding of just how damaging this natural and unconscious set of adaptive responses can be.

In 1956 Hans Selye published his studies of the effects of stress on health and on resistance to disease.[146] We now know that heart problems, high blood pressure, ulcers, arthritis, and other diseases are clearly connected to levels of tension and stress. The connections are easy to see, because we frequently feel the sensations associated with these problems at times of stress: the tightening of the muscles during an argument, the uncomfortable stomach before a difficult interview, the racing of the heart, sometimes a feeling of light-headedness. What isn't so obvious is that the effects of stress on the total system can create the conditions that lead to a much wider range of disorders than the ones we associate with those sensations.

Out of our individual experiences come habits and symbols. We react to situations in very direct ways, but we also *interpret* situations in the light of past experience, rightly or wrongly, and we react to those interpretations. A good part of our flexibility and our ability to anticipate trouble and prepare ourselves to deal with it before it happens depends on such interpretation, on recognizing situations where trouble might occur. The interpretation need not be verbal, or even conscious. The sight of a particular food that we have come to associate with a disgusting event can cause us to become nauseous. A dish that was served at a tense, unpleasant, but perhaps forgotten, meal long ago can spoil a marvelous meal for you today.

It isn't raw information that leads us to react in such specific ways. There is no such thing as raw information. We begin to interpret stimuli at the surface of the eye and the outer extremeties of the other senses, and we associate new information with past experience in subtle symbolic connections. We experience the world in a context of expectations, social demands, emotional states, habits of thought, and moment-to-moment needs and feelings. That context, coupled with the ways we have learned to interpret information, determines whether or not that information leads us to prepare ourselves for emergency.

Whether or not we actually do fight or flee in a given instance, whether or not our impulses to do so are translated into conscious action, the perceived and interpreted information produces detectable changes in the central nervous system. A complicated and wholly involuntary set of activities begins. When the hypothalamus receives the appropriate signal, the response takes place, whether you are facing a mugger, remembering being mugged, or simply worrying about being mugged. Any of these cases can initiate a response of equal intensity, and what is even more bothersome, your fight-or flight response might be triggered by passing someone on the street who is wearing the same sweater that you saw on a mugger, without it ever occurring to you consciously that the sweater is the reason for the reaction.

The hypothalamus, at the base of the brain—the same region that triggers the immune response—secretes substances that stimulate the pituitary gland, and this in turn secretes hormones that stimulate the appropriate endocrine glands. The chemical messengers roar through the bloodstream, setting us up for the burst of energy that a physical threat would necessitate. The endocrine glands secrete adrenalin and other hormones, which marshal our natural defenses to meet a challenge.

All of this may or may not be a response to an actual threat. It is a reaction to what is *interpreted* as a threat, and once it is begun it sustains itself. The arousal in the cortex, the action in the central nervous system, the secretions of the hypothalamus and the pituitary, the production of adrenalin, all enter into a great feedback loop. Once adrenalin is released into the bloodstream, accelerating heart action and setting the muscle tone, it triggers further responses in the hypothalamus. The increased muscle tension is added to the original perceived information and feeds back through the whole network once more as the blood pressure increases.

Hans Selye calls this the *general adaptation syndrome,* and in its extreme forms it allows us to deal effectively with emergencies. But suppose there is no real emergency to deal with? Or suppose it's not an emergency that we can deal with by either fighting or fleeing? Suppose we have to suppress the urge to release a sudden burst of energy? All that preparation to adapt ourselves to the needs of a threatening environment can turn back on us and damage tissue. In his more recent writings, Selye points out that many situations can trigger the stress response: extremes of heat or cold, illness, exertion, and even extremely *pleasant* situations. The response can be triggered *whenever we have to adapt and adjust to new situations*. And that is something that happens every day in many people's lives.

When stress is prolonged and the state of readiness is not discharged, the cortical hormones assume more importance. This is *chronic* stress. The feedback process, whereby the effects of one activity cause another, which then in turn reinforces the first, can lead to injury in the kidneys. The cortical hormones increase blood pressure, and at the same time they can cause damage to arterial walls, which is repaired by the kind of scar tissue called cholesterol placque. The control mechanisms in the liver, which normally regulate the level of cortical chemicals in the blood, are bypassed during stress, and the entire system runs amok. The cholesterol placques, which repair the arterial damage, can break loose and clog the arteries to the heart.

The study of stress has demonstrated that there is a clear connection between our states of emotional arousal and our states of health. Our *habits* of emotion, the ways in which we characteristically react to everyday situations, can make us prone to disease. Ulcers, nervous ailments, and cardiovascular disorders are easy enough to see in this connection, but it doesn't stop there. Rheumatoid arthritis, for example, seems to be influenced by emotion. Studies of the personal and emotional histories of people who contract the disease have established a picture of the arthritis-prone *personality*, something that mechanistic medicine couldn't have begun to talk about. According to the studies, people who are inhibited, self-conscious, conforming, compulsive, and capable of strong and rigid emotional control are the most likely to contract the disease.[156]

Preparing to deal with a situation that seems threatening, or to avoid it, or even to recover from dealing with it can *impair* our ability to cope with change by the very means designed to *help* us deal with it. We can make ourselves ill in the very process of adapting to changes in our daily lives.

Surveillance against Disease

What causes us to contract infectious disease? The easy answer, and the one we've become accustomed to, is that bacteria, viruses, and other foreign agencies invade our bodies and interfere with our natural functioning. In many cases we are able to throw off such diseases through the action of our own immune response, which maintains a constant surveillance over the human system and destroys foreign bodies which don't belong there.

As much as we like to think that we are the passive victims of virus infections, the viruses don't ordinarily appear and disappear in our surroundings at just the times we become ill. There is a fairly constant level of disease-bearing organisms around us all the time, and the sheer mobility of human beings increases the variety of such organisms that we come in contact with. If everything works properly, our immune systems provide us with effective defenses against the microbes. You "catch a bug," in most cases, when you let yourself become run down, over-tired, or depressed. It is common wisdom that we are likely to stay free of colds and flu if we keep our resistance high, maintaining a good state of health so that we can throw off the constantly present infectious organisms. And, with the exception of the particularly nasty viruses that are given such proper names as Asian Flu and Hong Kong Flu, most of us do succeed in throwing them off.

Now comes a sticky question: If the background organisms are always present and we contract illnesses for the most part only when our immune system is unable to deal with those organisms, then what *causes* the disease? This is like asking what caused Napoleon's defeat at Waterloo. Was it Wellington's strength or Napoleon's weakness? There are other difficult questions: What is the best way to treat such a disease? Should we try directly to wipe out the colony with antibiotics or other medications, or should we try to stimulate and enhance a person's own defenses against the established colony? Obviously, both approaches have value, and both should be used as we judge appropriate in specific cases. Antibiotics and other medications often produce side effects: destruction of healthy tissue, interference with the "friendly" digestive organisms that are essential to our proper functioning, or unnecessary dependence on the medication itself.

How we adapt to specific changes in the world around us, the rate and type of reaction we have, can make the difference between sickness and health. Some adaptations are relatively unconscious, some are totally so, like the adaptation to the splinter, and some are voluntary and deliberate adjustments in our behavior. How effectively you cope, consciously and unconsciously, with the world around you just is your state of health or disease: they are one and the same. But we tend to forget that our understanding and interpretation of our own experiences determine in large measure what there is to cope with. Some of our reactions to changes are dependent upon our perceptions; others are not. You will react to the splinter even if you don't feel it. Your first awareness that you have a splinter might—and often does—occur hours or even days after you get it, when the natural reaction to the invasion becomes apparent. In other cases the perception comes at the same time as the adaptation: You remark that the room is cold at the same instant that your skin starts rising in goose pimples and you begin to shiver. In still other cases, such as the reaction to the thought of a potential mugger, the adaptation is relevant *only* to your perceptions; there may never be a mugger.

A balance of processes and activities in the human system needs to be maintained for our continued well-being. It has variously been called *homeostasis,* or the integrity of the *milieu interieur,* or just the overall equilibrium of the body. Adaptation consists of alterations—usually minor—in natural activities directed toward maintaining the equilibrium. Norbert Wiener, the theoretical physicist associated with studies of feedback and cybernetics, sums up the matter: "The apparent equilibrium of life is an active equilibrium in which each deviation from the norm brings on a reaction in the opposite direction, which is the nature of what we call negative feedback." [180]

The familiar comparison between the natural feedback mechanisms of the human system and the thermostat that controls your furnace is precisely to the point. One of the most noticeable unconscious processes of the human system is the maintenance of body temperature. Perspiration, changes in the amount of blood that circulates to specific parts of the body, shivering, goose pimples—all are part of the unconscious homeostatic activity that keeps the dynamic equilibrium between the person and the environment in balance.

It's easy to get carried away with the beauty and symmetry of our unconscious balancing reactions and suppose that we are somehow in a perfect equilibrium. But, as Rene Dubos observes, "perfect homeostatic reactions are probably the exception rather than the rule.''[48] The so-called *wisdom of the body* is an ancient wisdom, remember, and it is not always suited to the conditions under which we live our lives in the last quarter of the twentieth century.

The emphasis on our biological means for surveillance against disease doesn't mean, of course, that every time you are ill it can be attributed to the subnormal activity of your immune response or an exaggerated response to stress. Some disease-bearing organisms and some carcinogens are clearly strong enough to overwhelm even the most resistant of us. Some of the stress-producing situations of modern life are unavoidable. What this understanding of disease does mean is that we have to pay more attention than we have to our own natural defenses against disease, to ways of strengthening and stimulating those defenses, and to ways of avoiding having them overpowered by combinations of circumstances.

CHAPTER THREE

The Special Problem of Cancer

What Cancer Is

Cancer is not a single disease. It occurs in an almost limitless variety of forms. It can strike almost anywhere in the system because it is a disorder of the cells that comprise tissues, organs, and fluids. Every cell in the human system has a specific genetic code that governs its replication, the process by which cells reproduce themselves. The genetic code, contained in a molecule of DNA within the cell nucleus, is passed on to the new generation of cells, governing their structure, their function, and ultimately the creation of yet other generations of cells in the constant process of renewal.

What ties all the separate manifestations of cancer together is what they have in common: the genetic material of some cells is altered so that any offspring from those cells are mutations, abnormal cells, that pass their abnormality along to their successors. At the same time, the mutant cells and the colony of offspring become less susceptible to the controls that naturally govern normal cellular growth. The conditions under which normal cells cease to multiply simply do not apply to cancer cells. This deadly combination of abnormal growth plus unrestricted multiplication can, and often does, produce a tumor or neoplasm that is malignant, threatening to life.

Cancer stands to Western medicine in much the same way that energy—heat, light, electricity and radioactivity—stood to Western physics at the turn of the century. The orthodox approaches to disease don't work with cancer, any more than the orthodox approaches of Newtonian mechanics worked with energy. There are limited successes, but our inability to get a genuine grasp of the problem has led to a scientific crisis, both in ways of dealing with the disease and in the theoretical understanding that guides the search for new treatments. When the full attention of the scientific community was directed toward understanding energy, the result was a significant change in the very basis of theoretical physics. Concepts and techniques changed, and the character of scientific questions changed. All of science was affected. Attempts to deal with cancer are bringing about a corresponding change in medical theory and practice, and in the kind of question that is asked and answered by the human sciences.

Questions about cancer once centered around how abnormal tissue invaded the body. Now they center on two somewhat different problems: Why do we generate abnormal cells, and why do some abnormal cells establish colonies while others don't? The answer to the first question is complex. It is likely that we generate abnormal cells in small quantities all the time. In addition, carcinogens in the environment stimulate the production of abnormal cells. Such elements are always present to one degree or another: radioactivity, excessive exposure to sunlight, industrial dyes, soot, asbestos, certain foods and food additives, tobacco smoke, automobile exhausts, insecticides. The list seems endless.

There are also carcinogenic viruses. About a dozen have been identified in animals. Unlike the viruses that cause infections by invading and destroying cells, cancer viruses invade the very nucleus of a cell and alter its genetic structure, changing the characteristics of its offspring and creating the possibility of a colony of abnormal cells. Finally, there is a tendency to produce specific types of cancerous cells that is clearly inherited.[41]

Under the best of circumstances it is difficult for an abnormal cell to reproduce itself. The immune system ordinarily recognizes cells that don't belong and destroys them. In order for a mutant cell to survive and multiply, it must escape the defense system. This happens in several ways. In some cases the *antigens*, substances that stimulate the immune response, are too subtle or too weak to trigger the response.[65] In other cases abnormal cells are generated so rapidly and in such vast numbers under the stimulation of carcinogens that they overwhelm the defenses. The immune response itself may be weakened by other factors so that it cannot properly maintain the integrity of the cells. Some deficiencies of the immune system are hereditary, and this, as much as an inherited tendency to generate abnormal cells, may account for certain types of cancer running in families.[92] The strength of the immune system also affects the success of organ transplants. They are successful only when the immune system is weakened in such a way that the transplant will not be rejected by the system's natural defenses. Certain forms of cancer occur more often in such cases than they do in the overall population. The link between impaired immune responses and the incidence of cancer seems to be well established.

Because the cluster of diseases we call cancer has proven so difficult to deal with, almost no hypotheses about the causes and possible treatments of the disease are dismissed out of hand. Any clue is welcome. One line of attack is of course to develop a better understanding of the structure of cells and the genetic chemicals DNA and RNA which govern their repro- duction. Another is to identify and eliminate those factors in the environment that stimulate the production of abnormal cells. Still another is the direct study of the natural defenses of the human system, which can prevent the establishment of colonies of abnormal cells. Each line of research has produced promising results, and each has given researchers a better understanding of how to prevent diseases other than cancer. The more we find out about cancer, the more we find out about disease in general.

The Cancer Profile

Surprisingly little is known about what *triggers* the human system's natural defenses against abnormal tissue, what condi- tions of the system promote or inhibit the growth of such tissue, and what makes the defenses effective in some cases and not in others. One way to come to understand cancer and our defenses against it is to study people who contract the disease. What do cancer patients have in common? What do those who have recovered from the disease have in common?

The pattern that has emerged from studies of cancer patients is an important part of the argument for holism. What cancer patients have in common most of all, aside from the disease itself, are specific psychological characteristics and specific kinds of emotional history.

It is not at all surprising to discover that there are typical emotional patterns that can be detected in people after they have contracted cancer. Illness can alter the chemical balance of the system so as to affect a person's mood and outlook, and the cancer diagnosis itself has an additional emotional impact. What *is* surprising is that the connection between disease and emotional states can run in the other direction as well.

Studies of the lifelong emotional habits and personal histories of cancer patients have been carried out in increasing detail and on increasingly wider scales over the past fifty years. The pace picked up during the 1950s, and recently the research has become quite intense. To date, more than two hundred separate reports have been published in medical and psychiatric journals concerning the emotional characteristics and the patterns of behavior of cancer patients. In one well-known study, published in 1956.[97] 250 cancer patients were given psychological tests and psychiatric interviews. A group of people who were not cancer patients were tested in the same way. Specific kinds of interpersonal relationships were found in the life histories of 62 percent of the cancer patients, and in only 10 percent of the other group. Since 1956 the results have been borne out by many similar studies.[9, 169]

A surprisingly specific cancer profile emerged from the studies. The pattern is established early in life, before the age of fifteen. It is characterized by feelings of isolation, neglect, and despair, which are typically associated with the breakup of a family unit by divorce, death, or serious friction between the parents. The individual feels responsible for the breakup and feels rejected because of it. Relationships with other people are considered futile and threatening. As an adult, the individual establishes a strong, central relationship to a single person or institution (a spouse or a child, or perhaps a job). A vast amount of emotional energy is invested in this relationship, and every effort is made to preserve it. The individual in effect becomes "too good to be true" in the attempt to maintain a thoughtful, gentle, uncomplaining attitude that will not threaten the single relationship. Finally, and perhaps inevitably, the adult relationship breaks in the natural course of events. The close attachment is never replaced. The individual feels despair, isolation, and—echoing back to the childhood component of the pattern—loss of meaning and feelings of being unworthy to enter into human relationships.

The striking thing about this pattern is that "with a high degree of predictability, such individuals are found to succumb to cancer within six months to a year" after the adult relationship is broken.[124]

Before you start looking for this cancer profile in yourself or those around you, let me point out that the connection is not established as causal in any sense, and that it is far from inevitable. What is important is the particularly acute form of depression, isolation, and despair that arises in adulthood after this sort of emotional history. The childhood isolation sets the stage, the single central relationship raises a possibility of never feeling that despair again, and the breaking of that relationship renews and intensifies the despair.

As a pattern of life history, the cancer profile is not at all uncommon. What seems to be at stake in this pattern is the *will to live,* and the sense of one's own worth that goes with it. When a person's will to live hangs by the slender thread of a single relationship, it is very fragile indeed. Grief over the loss of that relationship can literally kill. Other systematic studies of the emotional characteristics of cancer patients reveal similar insights into the connection between long-range emotional habits and resistance to the disease. For example, in one early study psychological testing of cancer patients yielded predictions of the speed with which tumors would grow, with 78-percent accuracy.[20] The patients whose psychological tests showed defensiveness, depression, a sense that life was meaningless, and low energy were the ones whose tumors tended to grow rapidly.

If specific emotional characteristics are linked to the development of disease, you would expect to see clear-cut differences between the incidence of cancer in the overall population and the incidence among mental patients, where emotional characteristics are exaggerated. Sure enough. The overall incidence of death from cancer among mental patients in general is less than half that of the population at large, with the specific exception of patients diagnosed with paranoia, which can be understood as a gross exaggeration of the feeling of personal isolation. Among paranoid patients the incidence of cancer is *higher* than in the overall population.[81, 142]

Other studies have confirmed the link between exaggerated emotional states and the incidence of cancer or its rapid development once it is established. In some studies psychological tests are given at the time of the biopsy or other means of diagnosis. The correlation between an established emotional habit of depression and hopelessness and the presence of the disease is striking. Moreover, the self-effacing "prince of a fellow" syndrome, as it has become known in the field—where a person maintains a facade that is just too good to be true in order to mask feelings of unworthiness—is a good indicator of those patients who are likely to have rapid-growing tumors. Independent of the cancer studies, it is well known that depression both precipitates and can be initiated by specific and measureable states of the body. The delicate and finely balanced chemical interchanges in the brain and nervous system that are the manifestations of our emotional states can be altered by dealing with the depression, and they can in turn influence other physiological states.

Does depression *cause* cancer? The most reasonable answer is "No." A complicated set of conditions has to exist in order for a person to contract the disease at all and in order for the disease to progress rapidly. An important *part* of those preconditions is clearly linked to personality and emotion, and to particularly acute negative feelings. Just as our perceptions of specific situations can lead to the fight-or-flight response, they can also lead to an unconscious response that amounts to giving up the constant surveillance against disease. According to Dr. Jerome Frank of the Johns Hopkins University Hospital, depression may inhibit the action of the immune system.[58]

Drs. Carl and Stephanie Simonton sum up their own research and that of many others: "We can surmise that there are significant emotional aspects connected not only with the course of malignancy, but also with the onset of the disease."[1]

Recent experiments with laboratory mice show that the connection between emotional stress and disease is not peculiar to human beings. At Carleton University in Ottawa, Lawrence Sklar and Hymie Anisman injected mice with live cancer cells and subjected some of them to frightening electric shocks that they could not avoid. A second group of animals received shocks of the same duration and intensity, but these animals were given a way to cope, to avoid the shocks. A third group received no shocks at all. The group that was unable to cope with stress developed tumors earlier, the tumors grew faster, and the animals died sooner than the animals in the other two groups.[155]

Dr. Claus Bahnson, Professor of Psychiatry at Thomas Jefferson University School of Medicine, believes that by the mid-1980s it will be possible, by means of psychological screening prior to the onset of disease, to predict at least 50 percent of cancer victims. The exact nature of the connection between lifelong habits of emotion and the incidence of cancer remains to be explained in detail, but there is little room for doubt that such a connection exists.

Dealing with Cancer

A diagnosis of cancer has an enormous emotional impact. First is the immediate fear of death itself. In addition to the dread of protracted pain, some of the very emotions that characterize the cancer profile are reinforced and intensified by the news of a cancer diagnosis: despair, a negative feeling toward oneself and one's body, a sense of isolation from others. Beyond these reactions, many patients view the treatments that face them as a chamber of horrors. The three principal treatments for cancer—surgery, radiation and chemotherapy—are unpleasant prospects. Each poses threats of its own, and none guarantees recovery. The sense of hopelessness frequently becomes worse, and the progress of the disease can be very swift indeed once the diagnosis is made.

In surgery the aim is to remove the cancerous growth. If the tumor is a solid mass, confined to one area, surgical removal may result in a cure, provided that the entire colony of abnormal cells is removed. Because this level of thoroughness is difficult to attain and even more difficult to be certain of, surgery is typically followed up with either radiation treatment or chemotherapy.

The aim of radiation therapy is to destroy the nuclei of malignant cells so that they cannot multiply. The identified tumor and the surrounding tissue are subjected to intense radiation, which destroys both cancer cells and normal cells. The size of the area irradiated must therefore be limited, and so must the frequency with which radiation is administered.

Chemotherapy, which is best understood as an attempt to poison the cancer cells by interrupting their metabolism, is typically used in conjunction with surgery or radiation to kill off those cells that remain after the more drastic local treatments.

Chemotherapy is the only one of the three standard therapies that treats the entire system. Whereas surgery and radiation treat only the area surrounding a tumor, the toxic chemicals used in chemotherapy are disseminated throughout the system, in the hope of killing the mutant cells while inflicting minimal damage on healthy cells and tissue. The possible side effects of both radiation and chemotherapy are unpleasant: nausea, changes in skin texture, hair loss, a general weakening of the entire system. Worse yet, both treatments can weaken the natural immune response so that a person's own defenses against the disease cannot be brought into play effectively.

These primary means of attack on cancer are all directed at existing cancer tissue, and their aim is to destroy or remove tumors from the body. Coupled with a program of early detection and diagnosis, they can be effective in many cases. But it is enormously difficult to isolate cancerous cells and attack them. A single tumor may contain as many as 100 million cells. If a combination of surgery and chemotherapy, for example, is 99.99 percent effective in destroying such cells, that still leaves 10,000 malignant cells after treatment, and each of those 10,000 cells could continue to multiply.[92] Surgery simply cannot be performed at the cellular level. Radiation cannot pick out all of the cancer cells in the body or sort out the cancer cells from healthy cells. The toxic substances used in chemotherapy spread throughout the system, but again the treatment is not selective; it destroys healthy cells and tissue as well.

Immunotherapy

The only known means for distinguishing healthy cells from abnormal cells is through the immune response, which constantly checks the genetic credentials of cells and eliminates those that don't belong. No known medical treatment can be as selective or as thorough. Increasingly, medical research is concerned with treating the host, the human system, rather than directly attacking the unwanted guests, the abnormal tissue and infectious organisms.[48] Cancer is coming to be viewed less as a localized problem confined to specific sites of tumors; instead it is increasingly seen as a disorder of the entire system.

Around the turn of the century, William B. Coley, a New York physician who worked with terminal cancer patients, noticed that one of his patients, who had developed a skin infection on his face, began to recover from his neck cancer as he recovered from the skin infection. The tumor began to shrink. Other physicians had observed similar coincidental recoveries from infection and cancer, but no one understood why it happened. Coley tried to develop a procedure that would take advantage of whatever the connection might be. He prepared extracts from mixtures of bacteria, which came to be called "Coley's toxins," and injected his cancer patients with them. Typically, the patients became very ill, showing all the signs of severe infection: chills, fever, muscle pains. But in many cases the cancer tumors changed as the patient fought the bacterial infection. The tumors softened, reduced in size, and in many cases disappeared altogether, never to return. In other patients cancer recurred, and in some cases there was no change at all. But a significant number of Coley's patients recovered from cancer and remained well for decades.[43]

Coley's treatment received a fair amount of attention at the time. There were difficulties with it, of course. The severe symptoms brought on by the toxic injections were sometimes life threatening. The toxins themselves were poorly understood, and it was difficult for Coley and other researchers to maintain the appropriate potency from one batch to another. Beyond this, no one understood *why* the induced symptoms of bacterial infection produced such positive results. These are the familiar problems of any new procedure, and one would expect Coley's story to finish up with a huge effort in research and theory, to perfect the toxin extracts and determine how they worked against cancer. But that's not the way it happened. At about this same time, x-rays were introduced for the treatment of various diseases, and it was x-rays rather than Coley's toxins that became the subject of intensive research. Coley's work was generally dismissed.[116]

Only very recently has research resumed on techniques like Coley's: *immunotherapy,* which involves the artificial stimulation of the immune system. Coley's toxins are now known to have activated the immune system to fight the bacterial infection and the abnormal cancer tissue as well, primarily by stimulating the blood cells called *macrophages* to extraordinary activity.

Macrophages are "non-specific"; they come into play in the immune system when certain types of invading organisms resist the more typical antibodies that provide protection against specific kinds of bacteria and viruses. In such a case, where specific antibodies are of no avail, *cell-mediated immunity* begins to operate. The white blood cells called *lymphocytes* multiply rapidly and secrete substances called *lymphokines,* which in turn stimulate the macrophages, the clean-up crew of the blood system. Once stimulated, the macrophages sweep through the system, killing and ingesting any infectious agents, bits of foreign matter, disease-causing fungi, and most important of all, cancer cells.[92]

Researchers in the United States, Canada, and France are currently studying non-specific immunotherapy as a possible treatment for cancer. Whether immunotherapy alone will ever provide an effective treatment for most forms of the disease is still in question, but it promises to provide at least a technique that can be used in combination with radiation therapy, chemotherapy, and surgery as a means of destroying any cancer cells that remain after the more common treatments.

The unique feature of immunotherapy is that it enlists a person's own defenses against the disease, stimulates and engages them in the destruction and elimination of abnormal cells. If cancer develops because the immune system is either overwhelmed or weakened, then it would seem reasonable to attack cancer by stimulating the immune system to extraordinary measures.

Since about 1975, excitement has increased about the possibilities of using the natural body protein *interferon* to stimulate our natural defenses against cancer. The protein has been recognized for more than twenty years, but its role in the immune response is still not fully understood. Cells produce interferon when they are invaded by viruses, but the protein itself does not attack the virus. Rather, it spreads to adjacent cells and triggers activity there, increasing the production of other proteins, which stop the spread of the virus.[75, 110]

Experiments at Stanford University Medical Center have shown that introducing interferon into the system of a cancer patient with a slow-growing tumor can produce shrinkage of the tumor within thirty days.[108] Other studies are directed toward inducing the system to increase its own output of interferon rather than introducing it from the outside. Until very recently, the only known source of interferon was human white blood cells, which meant that blood donors had to be found and the protein extracted in a difficult, expensive process. But a new technique called "gene-splicing" has made it possible to induce bacteria to produce human interferon in a way that promises to bring down the cost and increase the availability of the treatment. The work with interferon, spurred on by the special problem of cancer, has implications for the treatment of other diseases. Used as a nasal spray, interferon seems to prevent the common cold. Research with animals indicates that it is also effective against rabies, hepatitis, encephalitis, and yellow fever.

Disease and Holism

If you are studying the mechanical disorders of a clockwork, you are not likely to ask very many questions about its history or about why it has the characteristics it has. You examine the mechanism itself and try to understand how the pieces fit together and operate on a day-to-day basis, and then track down exactly which piece has developed trouble, where the repair or replacement has to be done. How this particular mechanism fits in with the rest of the world, or how it came to be the way it is, doesn't seem very important. You correct disorders at precisely the places where they show up.

The orthodox human sciences in general, including psychology, sociology, and anthropology, as well as medicine, have in the past taken the view that human beings are separate from the rest of nature and can be understood in isolation from nature. As Robert Ardrey and Konrad Lorenz have both argued, it is a mistake to assume that such a discontinuity exists between human beings and other animals, and between human beings and the environment that has made us the way we are.

The immune system isn't something that was developed yesterday to deal with the threats to human well-being that are common to twentieth century life. Biological development doesn't happen that way. Our natural defenses against disease are no more changed since the Stone Age than are our nutritional needs or our innate tendency to prepare ourselves to fight or flee when we are in a threatening situation. Understanding our own nature means understanding our biological history so that we can enlist our natural abilities in the attempt to maintain health under the conditions of modern life.

Beyond seeing ourselves as part of nature, we must come to a better understanding of the relationships between our emotional habits and our overall state of health. Selye's work on stress opens the door to questions about more subtle connections between the way we understand a situation and how we react to it physiologically. The emergence of the cancer profile raises even more general questions about long-term emotional habits and the ability of the whole human organism to cope with disease through the action of the immune system.

These distinctly holistic lines of inquiry should not be put into a false conflict with more traditional approaches to cancer and other diseases. We have to broaden the scope of medical questions, not abandon one approach in favor of the other. We need to know about the minute details of immunity and cell replication *and* about the limits of the whole organism's ability to deal with infection and mutant cells. Neither the study of cellular events nor the study of the larger relationships between the human organism and its surroundings will alone tell us what we need to know. We need to understand what the connections are between what we experience and the complex unconscious activities that are our reactions to experience.

As we see ourselves less in mechanical terms and more in biological terms, additional connections will begin to appear. And as we think of ourselves more in holistic terms, new questions can be asked about the kinds of conscious and unconscious activity that influence a person's state of health.

CHAPTER FOUR

The Will to Live, the Will to be Healthy

Directing the System's Defenses

Is there a day coming when cancer can be cured without surgery, without the horrors of chemotherapy or intensive radiation? Probably. But that day hasn't come yet. Cancer has resisted the approaches to prevention, treatment, and cure that have proven effective with other diseases, and for this reason researchers have tried new angles of approach. Some experimental techniques have had promising, even exciting, results, and they suggest ways in which medicine might deal with other kinds of illness as well as with cancer. But they are just beginning to come under serious clinical study. There is no "miracle cure" that anyone is sure of, despite the occasional rumors that one has appeared. Nothing has yet been found that is known to be as effective as surgery, radiation, and chemotherapy in one combination or another.

In treating a patient with an experimental technique, a physician is obligated by his professional ethics, by any reasonable set of personal morals, and by the law, to give the patient the most reliable and appropriate *known* kind of treatment before trying something that is not known to be effective. Experimental treatments have to be considered as adjuncts to more familiar medical techniques, until and unless enough evidence accumulates to justify considering some of them as genuine alternatives.

Since 1972 there has been considerable interest in the work of Dr. O. Carl Simonton, a radiologist who specializes in the treatment of tumors, and his wife, Dr. Stephanie Matthews Simonton, a psychiatric social worker. Their research has centered on cancer patients who defy the odds, those whose disease remains stable for a long period, or those who have complete remissions. The questions, of course, are what special characteristics set these "exceptional" patients apart from the rest, and how those characteristics can be passed along to other patients. The Simontons observed, as other clinicians had before them, that there seemed to be a common psychological thread that tied together those cancer patients who responded particularly well to treatment. In each case history it was noted that the person had a noticeably positive attitude toward the prospects for recovery from the disease and toward life in general. The *will to live,* which folk medicine and old-country grandmothers knew all about, assumed a new role in modern medical research.

The exceptional cancer patients were scrappy, determined people, who were self-reliant and inclined to take control of situations, including their own illnesses. Many of them had not only sought out the best traditional medical treatment, but they had also investigated less conventional treatments. They demanded information about the nature of the disease, and they were determined to be in charge of their own medical treatment and recovery.[1] The Simontons began to look for a way to *teach* this attitude to other patients. But how do you instill a positive attitude toward life and the prospects of recovery in a patient who is already depressed and overwhelmed by the news that he has cancer? How do you help such a patient relax and be confident that he can overcome cancer?

The Simontons studied "mind control" techniques to see if there was a way to generate in other cancer patients the characteristics that were typical of the "exceptional" patients. In 1971 Dr. Carl Simonton assembled a set of techniques to try with cancer patients who were referred to him for radiation therapy. He describes his work with the first patient:

> *In addition to the medical treatment, I explained to him what my thinking was. I told him how, through mutual imagery, we were going to attempt to affect his disease. He was a 61-year-old gentleman with very extensive throat cancer. He had lost a great deal of weight, could barely swallow his own saliva, and could eat no food. After explaining his disease and the way radiation worked, I had him relax three times a day, mentally picture his disease, his treatment, and the way his body was interacting with the treatment and the disease, so that he could better understand his disease and cooperate with what was going on. The results were truly amazing.[152]*

Amazing indeed! After three months of treatment, the patient recovered completely. A year and a half later, there was no sign at all that he had ever *had* throat cancer. This same patient, a feisty and funny gentleman, applied the technique himself to two other things that had been bothering him:

arthritis and impotence. He overcame both in the course of his daily exercises in visual imagery.

Such an incident could easily enough be dismissed if it were an isolated case. There are so many unknown factors in cancer, and in arthritis and impotence, for that matter, that any one of a number of things might have coincided with the long, intense period of relaxation and imagery. But it isn't an isolated case. Since 1971 Simonton has treated many cancer patients in this way, while of course simultaneously continuing more traditional treatments.

Simonton reports a case of a 33-year-old woman who was diagnosed as having cancer of the cervix. She refused the usual surgery, which involved removal of the uterus. She had been practicing meditation for some time, and under Simonton's direction she began meditating almost constantly, over a period of months, inducing a self-hypnotic state in which she visualized "a normal, healthy, beautiful uterus." Less than a year after the intensive self-hypnosis began, she was examined again. No trace of the cancer was found.

An Air Force pilot, near death and under treatment for advanced throat cancer, was taught by Simonton to induce an "alpha" state, a measurable condition of bioelectrical activity in the brain that is associated with overall relaxation. The nature of his disease was fully explained to him. He chose a visual imagery in which the defending white cells were "cowboys" on horseback, attacking and destroying cancer cells pictured as "bandits." The procedure was followed three times a day for fifteen minutes each time. After ten weeks the tumor (which had been the size of a peach) had receded and could not be detected. A biopsy of the patient's throat showed only normal tissue.

Reports such as these would have been considered an embarrassment to scientific medicine a few years ago. Trickery, misleading clinical conditions, or just plain bad science would have been suspected immediately. Few medical people would have thought it plausible that a technique like Simonton's could be effective. But conceptions have changed. Many physicians and psychologists around the country have begun to try such procedures as adjuncts to standard cancer treatments. The evaluation of such persuasive strategies will be difficult, but the experimentation and the ensuing critical dialogue indicate that the medical community is willing to take holistic approaches to disease seriously.

Dr. Neil Fiore, a psychologist who has cancer, has used Simonton's imagery technique and other psychological approaches to enhance the traditional cancer therapies he has received. He writes in the *New England Journal of Medicine* that therapists should encourage patients to attitudes of "exuberance, independence and individual responsibility," rather than keeping them sedated. "The patient's mental image of his or her disease and body can, through the workings of ideomotor responses, influence the direction of the body toward health or disease."[56]

In order to see that the Simontons' strategy is a plausible approach to cancer, we have to look at it a little more closely. Effectively, what Simonton's patients do is show themselves mental cartoons in which their own defenses win out over the manifestations of the disease. One patient visualizes the white blood cells as angry watchdogs chasing and attacking the cancer cells, which are visualized as masked vandals. Another visualizes the radiation as consisting of tiny bullets that hit all the cells in the area of the tumor. The normal cells repair the small amount of damage done, but the cancer cells don't. The white blood cells, the clean-up crew, transport the dead cancer cells through the bloodstream, liver and kidneys, and flush them down the urinary drain.

It isn't just a matter of making up a visual action sequence and thinking about it regularly. The patient is made to understand the nature of the disease and the treatment he has been receiving, and to understand the *conflict* between his own system and the disease. The conflict, which the good guys always win, is represented in the imagery. And to set the stage for the imagery, a suggestible state is induced by self-hypnosis, meditation, or one form or another of alpha-induction. The situation is established for the patient to "believe" in the cartoon drama between the representation of his natural defenses against disease and the representation of the disease itself. It isn't literally a matter of belief, of course; it is more like the special sort of belief you have when you really get involved in a play or a movie to the extent that you care about what is represented dramatically and respond emotionally.

Of course there is more to it than vivid imagery. The patients are given psychotherapy, along with their families when possible. Remember the cancer profile described earlier: the cycle of depression, self-dislike and pessimism that is statistically so prevalent in cancer patients, and *absent* in the exceptional cases the Simontons studied at the outset, has to be broken. The stage has to be set for successful treatment. If negative emotions can make one prone to cancer, then salutary emotions (Simonton calls them "welfare" emotions) may be a key to recovery.

Simonton believes that the real hero of the story is the immune system. Persuasive strategies of this sort may offset the weakening of the immune system that results from irradiation and chemotherapy, and tip the balance in favor of recovery. It is possible that such strategies might even be able to trigger the especially energetic activity of the immune response that figured in Coley's early procedures for immunotherapy.

The manipulation of perceptions and emotional states must either stimulate the immune system itself to extraordinary action, or overcome some of the factors which prevent the immune system from doing its job at specific sites. So the line of reasoning runs something like this: if the immune system is inhibited by depression (and there is plenty of evidence that it is, independent of Simonton's work),[58] then we should fight the depression with everything we have in the psychological arsenal. *Believing* in the representations of disease and defending white blood cells, and *believing* that the white blood cells can and do win out, with as much intense involvement as you've ever experienced at a movie or a play, and perhaps more, can influence your mood and outlook. If you could view that movie three times a day, every day, with the same degree of involvement, the positive and optimistic mood and outlook would become pretty much of a habit. The use of hypnosis, meditation, or the alpha state makes the intense involvement with the vivid images possible. And that in turn produces a general state of "welfare" emotion. Simonton believes that the overall positive emotional state leads to a general stimulation of the immune system, which then attacks the abnormal cells with greater vigor.

But is there more to it than that? Do the vivid images somehow *direct* the body's defenses to take extraordinary measures at specific sites? Almost every medical writer who has heard of Simonton's work has a pet hypothesis as to how the visual imagery and the associated techniques affect the disease. It seems plausible that these patients are really taking over the direction of the immune system, sending it messages. One prominent medical writer has even suggested that what is involved is related to *psychokinesis,* the ability to move objects just by deciding to.[119] But we know less about such "psychic" phenomena than we know about cancer, and it is neither necessary nor appropriate to turn in that direction for an explanation of the success of persuasive strategies like Simonton's. There are far more plausible explanations to be had.

We can't destroy cancer calls *just* by deciding to, or cure arthritis or other ailments. Our unconscious activities, the things we do in our bloodstream and glands, don't respond to direct commands as a rule. But they do respond to cues and messages that are something other than direct commands, and those cues can be deliberately manipulated. It involves a bit of trickery.

Think of the production of saliva. Under ordinary circumstances, we produce saliva at a given "resting" rate all the time. But under specific stimulation, in anticipation of food, like Pavlov's dogs, we salivate at a much higher rate. Can you *make* yourself salivate at the higher rate at will? Of course you can, but if you are like most people, you can't do it just by deciding to. Typically, you can trigger the higher rate of saliva production by thinking about food—especially if you think about foods that you like, and *most* especially if you intend to have some of that food at a definite time in the near future. Think about your favorite dinner. Imagine it laid out before you. Decide right now to have it tomorrow evening. Believe that you will. Now imagine yourself savoring each mouthful. It works, doesn't it?

Now what happened? You deliberately tricked yourself into a bit of ordinarily automatic behavior, the production of a high level of saliva; and you used imagery to do it. The more vivid the imagery, the more saliva you probably produced.

To view this as a case of "mind over matter" is just misleading. There aren't *two* things involved here, a mind-thing and a body-thing. There is just *one* thing: a person, a whole functioning organism, performing one sort of activity consciously in order to be able to perform another sort of activity that is not totally conscious.

Simonton's work bears out what other researchers have detected about the relationship between mood, attitude, and emotion on the one hand and the functioning of the immune system on the other. But it raises some really interesting questions, too. To what extent can we deliberately contrive ways to influence our involuntary activities? If we can unwittingly make ourselves ill by means of perceptions and emotions, can we also promote healing in this way? Can we improve our overall health through such means even in the absence of disease?

Sending Ourselves Messages

"We are sending ourselves messages all the time. We maintain a running dialogue with ourselves. Depression is a message, and all too often it is a message that we respond to in very direct ways." The speaker is Dr. Clorinda Margolis, of the Department of Psychiatry and Human Behavior at Jefferson Medical College in Philadelphia. She is known to the cancer patients in the wards as the "hypnosis lady," who helps them to overcome pain.

Hypnosis, in one form or another, has been used to relieve pain for perhaps thousands of years. But despite many attempts over the past few centuries to develop regular, recognized clinical procedures which included hypnosis, it was not acknowledged as a legitimate medical tool by the American Medical Association until 1958.

It is now a familiar matter in many hospitals to see a psychologist sitting by the bed of a patient with intractable pain, speaking gently in a slow, repetitive monotone, asking the patient to remember a peaceful scene, or to fix attention on a watch or a pendulum until the patient's eyelids become heavy. Sometimes the patient will be asked to count, forward or backward, or to imagine slowly descending a staircase, or to develop his own associations and images of a peaceful, relaxed situation. Gradually, working with the patient's own images, the psychologist suggests descent, downward motion, and greater relaxation at each step. With patients who are experienced, he may simply give a few cues or ask the patient to put himself into an "alpha state" or to meditate.

The guidance and suggestion can take several forms. Some patients are open to hypnosis and will respond quickly to the direct suggestion of numbness or absence of pain in the affected area. Others will respond only if there is a reason suggested for the numbness: They are asked to imagine that a local anesthetic has been injected, or that the nerves in the affected area are controlled by switches in the brain, which they can turn off at will. According to a standard medical text on the subject, "The highly hypnotizable person finds this exercise of imagination entirely congenial; the less hypnotizable finds in it a way of directing his effort toward control."[74] With a new or skeptical patient, some explanation is usually necessary, perhaps some reassurance that nothing magical or unnatural is going on.

If the direct suggestions or the images of switching off pain are not effective, other methods are tried. For example, "Glove anesthesia" develops a feeling in the hand of heat or cold, or that the hand is made of wood, or that a protective glove has been drawn on. Suggestions of drastic changes in temperature, as if the hand were in very hot water or in ice water, or holding a snowball, often produce numbness or local anesthesia and at the same time alter the measurable flow of blood to the hand. The message from the stimulated imagination gets through to physiological activities. It sometimes takes a demonstration that the imagination *can* be stimulated to affect pain before a patient will be successful. Once glove anesthesia is mastered, the patient can often extend the procedure to other parts of the body.

In other cases the pain can be "converted" to a pleasant tingling sensation. In still others, the pain can be displaced from one part of the body to another, so that severe abdominal pain will seem to be in the hand rather than in the abdomen.

The displacement might take the form of locating intense pain spatially within the body and then diffusing it throughout the entire body, with a corresponding lessening of intensity. Increasingly, hypnotic treatment for pain is turned over to the patient, who is taught and encouraged to practice the relaxation and the imagery several times a day.

The reasons why this technique hasn't been available before or been seriously studied until the past twenty or thirty years go back to the familiar commitments of mechanistic science. An enormous amount of unscientific lore has always been associated with hypnosis. It was part of the alien tradition of Eastern science, which has traditionally been suspect in the eyes of Western researchers. Moreover, hypnosis was often associated with wandering quacks and healers. It had religious, mystical, theatrical, and magical connotations, which excluded it from serious scientific consideration. And worst of all, hypnosis seemed to involve a mental cause for physical events, something no self-respecting Newtonian scientist would consider seriously.

The first recorded attempt to bring the phenomenon into the arena of Newtonian science came with Franz Anton Mesmer's publication of his theory of ''animal magnetism'' in 1774. Mesmer and other researchers became interested in hypnosis because it apparently brought relief from pain and some specific symptoms of disease. Mesmer believed that the most important element in the hypnotic transaction was the hypnotist's power, not the subject's receptiveness. His public demonstrations were marvels of showmanship, and they served to reinforce Mesmer's own belief that in hypnosis some *force* passes between one person and another. ''Forces,'' radiant energy of any sort, posed a difficulty. Any explanation of a transfer of energy had to obey the rules of Newtonian science, and the most important rule of all was that every natural process was mechanical. Heat and light had been

understood since Newton as consisting of either minute cor-
puscles of matter or as "subtile fluids" that pervaded all space.
When the French chemist Lavoisier, in the eighteenth century,
tried to describe the chemical nature of matter and to determine its basic constituents, it was perfectly reasonable for him
to treat both heat and light as chemical elements, "substances"
whose particles interacted mechanically with the particles of
other substances.

No wonder, then, that Benjamin Franklin's theory of electricity, put forward in the 1740s and still defended a hundred
years later, identified electricity as a fluid that was present in all
matter. An object with more than what Franklin called its
natural share of electricity was positively charged; an object
with less was negatively charged. Any electrical activity consisted, literally, of the flow of the electric fluid from the object
with more than its natural share to the object with less, and this
flow was to be understood according to the mechanical principles of hydrodynamics.[157]

Mesmer's explanation of the supposed hypnotic force had
to conform to the same scientific rules. Like Franklin and
Lavoisier, he developed a theory that postulated a peculiar
kind of fluid, a magnetic fluid that pervaded all matter but was
particularly concentrated in living beings. He claimed that
many forms of illness could be understood as the result of a
lack of the magnetic fluid. The hypnotist (the "magnetizer" in
Mesmer's terms) was able to relieve the symptoms of migraine,
hysteria, and arthritis because the subtle fluid passed invisibly
from the magnetizer to the patient, in much the same way that
Franklin's electric fluid was understood to pass from one object
to another. There was some question whether the magnetizer
was the source of a superabundance of the magnetic fluid or
merely a channel directing the fluid from some outside source.

This isn't the crackpot idea of an 18th-century confidence
man. Mesmer's theory, like Franklin's, was in the best tradi-

tion of the mechanistic understanding of energy. It wouldn't have occurred to him or to anyone else at the time to look for a psychological explanation for the relief of physical symptoms. Any treatment that had a positive effect on physical illness had to be understood as a direct mechanical intervention in the malfunctioning of a physical system.

The controversy over Mesmer's work led the king of France to appoint a commission in 1784 to study hypnosis and Mesmer's theory explaining it. The members included Ben Franklin himself, the chemist Lavoisier, and the physician and inventor Dr. Joseph Guillotin. Their aim was to determine whether or not Mesmer really had discovered a new physical fluid that would take its place beside heat and electricity. The study of the medical effects of the technique was secondary. The commission concluded that no independent physical evidence of the magnetic fluid could be produced apart from the claimed cures themselves. They attributed the apparent therapeutic effects of the technique to imagination and suggestion. There was no need, of course, to explain *how* imagination and suggestion could function to alleviate genuine bodily symptoms. They couldn't; not if the body was a machine. Any symptoms relieved by hypnosis had to be bogus to start with.[61]

Medical researchers continued to be fascinated by hypnosis, but the royal commission's verdict discouraged any further work with the technique. In the 1840s the Scotch surgeon James Esdaile carried out 300 major surgical operations in India using "Mesmeric trance" as the sole anesthesia, but the medical journals of his day refused to print his findings. British physicians of the same period who used hypnosis in amputations were called liars by the Royal Medical and Chirurgical Society.[89] Just as the rise of radiation therapy led to the relative neglect of research in immunotherapy eighty years ago, the introduction of ether in 1846 and chloroform in 1847 weakened the arguments for studying hypnosis as a surgical anesthetic. Since hypnosis didn't fit the "model" for a proper medical technique, the practice of surgery under hypnosis and the interest in the field became less widespread once chemical anesthetics were available.

Throughout the 19th century and into the 20th, only a few maverick researchers worked with hypnosis, and not many of them kept their ties with the medical profession. In 1895, when Freud and Joseph Breuer became convinced that hypnosis was a reliable tool for the treatment of hysterical patients, it became associated almost exclusively with psychoanalysis and psychotherapy; but even there it disappeared from the mainstream. After World War I, and again after World War II, hypnosis was used widely in the treatment of shell shock and battle fatigue. In the 1950s, the postwar interest in the technique caught hold, and the use of hypnosis as an anesthetic in dentistry, childbirth, and surgery began to increase. Hypnosis is now well established in both medicine and psychology, and funding and research facilities are available for studies of hypnosis and its applications which employ the same critical scientific methods used in the study of other clinical procedures. It is now established that hypnosis can relieve pain and suffering as well as other methods, and in some cases better.[74]

There are several competing theories about how hypnotic pain relief works. One theory suggests that hypnosis triggers either a natural "nerve block" or a reaction in the brain chemistry that releases natural opiates to lessen the transmission of pain signals along specific channels. In psychotherapy, hypnosis has been effective in bringing repressed memories to the surface, in helping patients whose interpretations of situations around them lead to phobias—fears of crowds, confined spaces, heights—and in breaking compulsions such as smoking.

But the fascinating part of hypnosis research, and the part that has more direct bearing on the turn to holism, is that clinicians are beginning to treat overt physical symptoms with hypnosis. It seems paradoxical that medical scientists have been saying for generations that religious "miracles" and cases of spontaneous bleeding and stigmata are, if not due to fakery, probably the result of hypnosis or self-hypnosis, while at the same time they refused to look seriously into the possibility of positive medical applications of the technique.

There are now well-tested and fairly predictable situations where hypnotic suggestion can be used to relieve psoriasis, an uncomfortable and unsightly skin disease,[61] and assist in the healing of wounds. In addition, as Lewis Thomas puts it, "Warts can be ordered off the skin by hypnotic suggestions."[171] Thomas, who is as cautious and conservative as any contemporary medical authority in accepting the claims of emotional influences on physiological disorders, describes the hypnotic removal of warts as "a wonderful problem, in need of solving," because warts are caused by a specific virus, and it is not at all well understood how hypnosis and imagery can make certain areas of the skin suddenly inhospitable to that virus.

Hypnosis can also be used to increase or decrease the flow of blood to specific parts of the body. In circulatory disorders such as Raynaud's Syndrome, or in migraine headaches, control of the flow of blood can provide relief that is unavailable with other methods of treatment. It has also been used with hemophilia, an inherited disorder in which the blood does not clot properly, to reduce the circulation of blood to the gums so that teeth can be pulled without precipitating heavy bleeding. At the Medical Center of the University of Colorado at Denver, hundreds of hemophiliac patients have been taught to induce hypnotic trance in order to control bleeding. Children as young as five are taught to "do trance" in order to draw blood to the fingers and toes and away from the joints, where painful and harmful bleeding often occurs under the skin. The constant fear of minor injury that has always limited the freedom of hemophiliacs can, with training, become a thing of the past. The technique must be practiced regularly, at least twice daily, like other hypnotic and meditative techniques. When it becomes a familiar part of the daily routine, "doing trance" can be called on in the event of injury, to reduce the severe bleeding that is the terror of hemophiliacs and their families.

It is cases like these that make you wonder just what the limits are for taking deliberate control of our unconscious activities. Some dramatic manifestations of physical symptoms that we associate with theatrical performances of hypnosis have now been repeated under experimental conditions. A hypnotized subject, told that his skin is about to be touched with a lighted cigarette, when it actually is touched with an ordinary pencil eraser, will develop blisters at the spot, as if he really had been burned. That is control of a sort that you might not particularly want to have, but it indicates that our natural and unconscious activities to deal with injury can be directed to specific sites by means other than the automatic reactions stimulated by the injury itself. It suggests that those startling imagery techniques of Simonton's might, indeed, bring about extraordinary activity at the site of cancer tumors.

Not everyone can be hypnotized, however. The susceptibility to hypnotic induction follows a "normal curve" over the total population. About 80 percent of the population is responsive to some degree. Similar curves describe the susceptibility of people to antibiotics and other drugs.

Current researchers do not share Mesmer's conviction that hypnosis involves an exchange of energy. The dominant theories now focus on the trance state itself. Research since 1959 indicates that the state can be self-induced, and that it sometimes happens spontaneously and unobtrusively when we are, for example, listening to music. According to one well-accepted description, hypnosis consists of the construction, either by the subject or by an operator (hypnotizer), of a special temporary orientation to a small range of preoccupations, coupled with the relative fading of awareness of the surrounding situation.[149,150] Reality doesn't slip away. It is voluntarily, deliberately, and temporarily suspended. What separates hypnosis from the relaxation techniques it resembles, such as meditation, is that once the trance state is reached the subject is more receptive to direct and indirect suggestion and imagery. The imagination can be directed toward specific goals.

The history of hypnosis in Western culture, its use in magic shows and the mysterious artifacts that have surrounded its use, distract us from the realization that the ability to enter the trance state and to bring about physiological changes by directing the imagination in specific directions is a part of human nature, just as much as the immune response or the fight-or-flight response are. The stress reaction—Selye's general adaptation syndrome—isn't unique and it isn't the only case where automatic, involuntary physiological changes can be initiated by the way we interpret specific situations, or even by memory or imagination. Once we come to understand our biological heritage better than we do now, we can learn to stimulate our natural responses, to manipulate them deliberately, to make them work for us rather than against us, in order to promote healing and maintain health.

Adaptation and Perception

The modern understanding of hypnosis provides some insight into how we can make ourselves ill as well as how we can cope with illness and pain. It shows just how explicit the messages we send to ourselves can be: that startling business of raising real blisters on the skin at the site of an *imaginary* cigarette burn sticks in the mind. It is clear that beliefs, suggestions, and expectations can and do alter measurable physiological states.

Clorinda Margolis tells of a saleswoman who complained

about the excessive air-conditioning in the store where she works. "I'm going to be sick tomorrow," she said. And of course she was. It was almost a statement of intention. Sometimes we can perversely will ourselves to be ill. In a similar case, a young opera student developed strep throats with uncanny timing a day or so before an important performance or audition. At lessons or rehearsals he was fine. If a performance or an audition came up without much warning, he would have the characteristic case of nerves but would deal with that and sing well. However, given a few weeks notice of an important performance, about two days before he was scheduled to go on, he would get a throat infection, complete with high fever and the classic white spots in the throat that often indicate strep infection. Throat cultures confirmed the diagnosis. Eventually, the young singer gave up performing altogether. Instead, he became a professional philosopher, and now writes books about changing concepts in the sciences.

Sometimes we deal with threatening situations by avoiding them, by giving ourselves an out. At one time or another, we have all known (or been) a person whose illnesses are so exquisitely timed to life's major and minor crises that there can be no doubt of the connection between the crisis and the illness. With that perfect timing, can we really believe that the illness isn't faked, as a means for dealing with a difficult situation? Of course, there are out-and-out fakes, the family tryants who directly threaten to have heart attacks if they don't get their way. That's not a medical problem, it's an ethical one. The trouble is, we often cannot be sure in such cases, not even about ourselves. We can trick ourselves into a genuine illness just as surely as we can trick ourselves into producing enough genuine saliva for a superb but imaginary meal.

A physician friend tells of his "anniversary syndrome." Every year, at about the same time, he develops an uncomfortable flu-like infection, combined with severe depression. Several years ago, he made the connection between the time of his annual illness and the anniversary of the death of his younger sister many years ago. But the annual illness happens even in years when he doesn't think of his sister's death. It's difficult to spell out clear distinctions in such a case because the "anniversary syndrome" is not an imaginary disease, any more than the singer's certifiable strep throat was. The symptoms are perfectly genuine, and they have a reality independent of the patient's perception of them. The suspicion is, however, that the disease is occasioned by the memory of an event, and in the singer's case by the dread of it. This is called a *psychogenic* disease.

In each example the patient made himself ill, but in a paradoxical way. It would be difficult to say that it was willful because it would seem to be *against* the patient's will. But where is the line drawn between a psychogenic disease and the obvious fakes who *threaten* to become ill? Do we ever willfully make ourselves ill? Sometimes, sure we do. The cancer profile is dynamite, and if we take it seriously, we have to ask some uncomfortable questions about whether we are always the victims of illness or sometimes bring it on ourselves. Until recently it has been easy to dismiss the question of responsibility. It *has* been a matter of folk medicine, old wives' tales, and unscientific lore that a connection exists between personality—which I prefer to think of as a person's emotional habits—and disease. But there is now enough hard experimental evidence for such a connection that it cannot be ignored.

It begins to sound as if every time we're ill, it's our own damned fault, either because we haven't taken care of ourselves, or because we sent ourselves the wrong messages. No; often we are simply overwhelmed by the conditions or the organisms that lead to disease. Proponents of holistic approaches to health are very sensitive to this matter of "blaming the victim." The combinations of circumstances known to lead to cancer and heart disease are complex, and it is generally impossible to reconstruct exactly why one person becomes ill and another doesn't. It is idle, in most cases, to ask whether a little less exposure to conditions that carry a risk of disease or a little more resistance to those conditions would have prevented the illness. But it isn't idle at all to attempt to minimize your exposure to risk conditions and at the same time to enhance your ability to deal with those that are unavoidable. If you are ill, you can improve your own ability to deal with the disease while still following the best available medical advice in treating it. Perceptions, emotions, and attitudes *are* involved in maintaining and recovering health. Taking responsibility for your own health includes coping with those factors as a matter of personal hygiene. Adaptation, which includes both the immune response and the stress response, happens at both conscious and unconscious levels. And in both cases it happens at least in part because of the way we perceive situations. Sometimes the stress created by overwhelming responsibility creates illness, and sometimes, as with students who are genuinely sick to their stomachs on the day of the big test, the illness is a clear response to a message; the message is "Run and hide."

A new direction is being taken in the study of perception, as well as in the study of how our perceptions can affect our health. Until recently research on perception, especially in this country, has concentrated on the physiological "mechanisms" of perception and the "processing system" in the brain and nervous system. The analogy between the human perceptual system and a digital computer took hold, and the assumption was that the "computer" in the human organism was unprogrammed, that perceptions were processed as raw data. Many psychologists have recently come to favor a *phenomenological* approach to perception, which allows us to pay more attention to the way we react to complex and meaningful stimuli. Our present experiences are interpreted in the context of our expectations (remember the mugger) and our past experience. Our perceptions of things and events around us are integrated into a personal frame of reference that includes ourselves and our expectations, our knowledge and beliefs, our hopes and the things we dread. At present there is little constructive theory about the *way* in which perceptions are integrated into individual frames of reference. The direction is pointed for a new psychology of perception, but the serious work has just begun.[176] Now that there is good reason to believe that our perceptions are of direct medical relevance to the onset of disease and the recovery from it, you can be sure that the critical scientific debate over the psychology of perception will heat up over the next several years.

All of this stimulated activity within the human sciences is the direct result of a particularly holistic insight: The state of your health, good or bad, is the result of the complex interaction of social and emotional factors, the conditions and pace of your life, physical and psychological stress, your perceptions of the world around you and the events that take place in that world, and your reaction to those perceptions. Your own ability to adapt adequately to the circumstances of your life in both conscious and unconscious ways is probably the most crucial single influence on your health.

CHAPTER FIVE

Medical Intervention

The shift to a holistic point of view on medicine and health involves more than specific new developments in therapeutic technique; it also involves new bases for making judgments about the best way to intervene in the course of established disease. There are honest arguments within the medical professions about the effectiveness of what has come to be called "orthodox" Western medicine. For a person with a serious illness, this can be demoralizing, especially when the argument isn't about which surgical procedure or medication to use, but about whether surgery or medication is called for at all, beyond those measures which directly aid the system in combatting the illness.

Many medical critics complain that traditional Western medicine prefers to take more extreme measures than the illness calls for; that surgery is performed simply because surgery is possible; that we over-medicate ourselves, and substitute medication for common sense. To some extent, the criticisms are justified. But on the other hand, most of us would hate to be in a situation where the advanced techniques of modern surgery and medicine were unavailable when we really needed them. That's the question, then: When are dramatic interventions called for, and when is it more appropriate to intervene in much less dramatic and immediate ways by sensibly changing the circumstances and habits of a person's life that have brought about the disease?

There is no easy answer, and no simple formula can be applied in all cases. Beware of what Lewis Thomas calls "Magic in Medicine": the often simplistic attribution of all human ills to the presence or absence of some particular substance in the diet, the claims of universal cure-alls, or the idea that some particular program of personal habit can guarantee everyone a long and healthy life with no need for medication, surgery, or other treatment.[171] Reality just isn't that simple; our knowledge of the causes and the most effective treatments of specific illnesses is limited by the evidence that is available to us at any given time.

One of the major benefits of holism is that it increases the medical options. There is no reason to *exclude* any established approach to treatment. But holistic approaches to treatment may provide alternatives to more traditional measures in many cases, and future research that is influenced by holism is bound to uncover even more alternative ways to deal with a given disorder.

Surgery

The drastic and dramatic techniques that have been developed for dealing with emergencies and for repairing damage at specific sites are unique to modern Western medicine. They would probably never have been developed were it not for the mechanistic commitments that I've been contrasting to holism. The very idea of opening up the body, fixing what's wrong, and sewing it up again is as mechanistic as can be. It resembles the way we take care of a malfunctioning automobile or toaster.

Many medical authorities believe that surgery is too often

relied upon as the first line of defense, especially against cardiovascular diseases, when it should be resorted to only when all else has proven ineffective. Surgery has become something of a habit with Americans over the past few generations. The "I-break-it-you-fix-it" relationship between patient and surgeon is under fire, with both patients and physicians being admonished to put prevention before repair, and to put nonsurgical medical treatments before surgery whenever possible.

According to figures released by HEW, 2.83 million unnecessary surgical operations were performed in the United States in 1974, at a cost of $3.92 billion. Between 1970 and 1975 the number of surgical operations increased by 23 percent, four times greater than the growth of the population. For both medical and economic reasons, medical associations, government agencies, and insurance companies are urging people to seek a second opinion when a physician recommends surgery.

There is growing controversy within the medical profession concerning specific surgical procedures. The coronary bypass operation for angina pectoris and myocardial ischemia is a case in point. Angina pains result from the occlusion or partial blockage of an artery that supplies the heart muscle with blood. The surgeon removes a piece of vein from the patient's leg and uses it to bypass the occluded part of the coronary artery, thereby restoring an adequate supply of blood to the heart muscle. The relief from pain is often immediate and dramatic.

New surgical procedures such as the coronary bypass can come into general and widespread use without animal or human testing, without formal experimental designs to demonstrate their effectiveness, and without long-term follow-up investigation.[26] Drugs, of course, are subject to such testing, and there are routine follow-up procedures to determine their long-range effects. But with surgery, physicians and surgeons operate more autonomously and independently than they do with other procedures. They do not regularly share information or compare their experiences with patients. Since the coronary-artery bypass graft was introduced in 1969, more than 250,000 patients have had the operation; more than 80,000 Americans underwent the operation in 1978 alone.[62] There is no way to tell about the quality of life that follows such surgical intervention. The one important study that has been published[114] involved 600 patients who received the procedure under experimental conditions, and a good amount of controversy has arisen concerning the study. For the majority of the patients studied (with the exception of those whose left main artery was involved), there was no difference in the survival rate between patients who received only medical treatment and those who had the surgery, and there was no measurable physiological difference between the two groups either. The operation does bring significant relief from pain, however, and this has been the main argument in its favor. But there is no means for following up the effect on the overall quality of life in those 250,000 patients who have had the bypass operation, and this blunts the arguments on both sides.

Other arguments have arisen concerning "routine" surgical procedures that are inherently dangerous, and that have not been demonstrated to be more effective than non-surgical measures. Radical mastectomy is the most widely used operation for breast cancer, for example, even though there is strong evidence that it is no more effective in prolonging life and relieving symptoms than simpler procedures. Even the old-fashioned tonsillectomy, which used to be routine for children, has been questioned. Strong indications exist that the long-term incidence of throat infections is no greater in people who keep their tonsils, yet one million tonsillectomies are still performed annually in this country.[62] We have been taught to believe in surgery, and not even the strongest critics would argue that surgery is *never* called for. The criticism centers on the headlong rush to surgery before other treatments have been considered.

For coronary occlusion the alternatives to surgery are more diffuse, less dramatic, and less obviously decisive, even though evidence shows that they are just as effective clinically. The use of drugs that affect the heart by reducing the work it must do, or by blocking the receptors of adrenalin that accelerate heart rate, is not nearly so convincing to the patient as the high drama of open-heart surgery. The insistence that the patient must change the lifestyle which brought about the disorder in the first place seems tiresome and tedious to many patients, and too "ordinary" a measure to be effective. Rather than reducing weight, cutting out smoking, controlling diabetes, modifying the diet, increasing exercise, and taking steps to lower the cholesterol level, many patients and physicians seem to prefer to get it over with in one dramatic surgical move. Many physicians regard surgery as the only "rational" procedure, the only remedy where straightforward cause-and-effect relationships can be seen. Techniques considered to be apparently "irrational" for relieving pain are effective in about 50 percent of patients with arterial placques, however.[122] And since it is the relief of pain which is advanced as the strongest argument in favor of the surgery, it may be that we need to revise the notion of what is and what is not a "rational" procedure.

The evidence is increasing that surgery is effective in many cases simply *because we believe in it.* Dr. Jerome Frank, one of the most vocal critics of a total reliance on mechanistic intervention, suggests that an attitude of "expectant faith" is extremely powerful, that "the state of mind engendered by the operation" can often be more effective than surgery itself. About the coronary bypass, Frank states: "The surgeon almost literally kills the patient and then resurrects him. Very few faith healers can make such an impressive demonstration."[59]

Somewhat waggishly, Frank suggests that hospitals represent healing shrines to modern Americans; that faith in "St. Johns Hopkins" is as effective in working miracle cures at that hospital as it is at any religious shrine:

Let's try to imagine, if you will, how Johns Hopkins might look to an anthropologist who knew nothing of the science of medicine and had heard that Hopkins was a healing shrine and was studying it from this aspect. He would learn that first of all it had an immense reputation as the site of miraculous cures. And he would be impressed with the massive, labyrinthian buildings situated on a hilltop, through whose many orifices pilgrims seeking health are continually streaming. Inside he would find a complex structure, with certain areas open to the public, such as the wards, and others where members of the staff perform mysterious healing rituals and to which they alone have access, such as laboratories, operating rooms, radio-therapy rooms, and intensive care units. These rooms contain spectacular machines which beep and gurgle and flash lights, or emit immensely powerful, invisible healing rays, thereby impressively invoking the healing powers of science. The operating rooms of course are the holy of holies, where the most dramatic and difficult healing rituals are conducted. Even the priests can enter only after donning special costumes and undergoing purification rites known as scrubbing. So jealously guarded are the mysteries of the operating room that patients are rendered unconscious before entering them. Our anthropologist would note that the organization of St. Johns Hopkins is highly structured, each echelon having its own insignia of rank and function. All members of the priesthood speak to each other in an arcane language, unintelligible to the layman, and prominently display on their persons healing amulets and charms, such as reflex hammers, stethoscopes and ophthalmoscopes. At the lowest level are the postulants in their short white jackets; above them the acolytes, who wear white suits, and above them the priests, especially impressive in their long, white, starched coats. All are expected to dedicate themselves to the service of the shrine, regardless of personal hardship or interference with connubial felicity and other satisfactions of life.

Well, let me come back down to earth after that flight of fancy and remind you that the powerful influencer of the patient's psychic state is the physician, whose power comes from two sources at least. The first is that he occupies a social role of respect and trustworthiness analogous to that of a parent, so he mobilizes the attitudes of trust and dependency that an infant feels toward a good parent. Secondly, his treatment is validated by a theory which both expresses and confirms the world view of the society in which both he and the patient function. Since a shared world view both makes sense out of life and reinforces the sense of group belongingness, medical treatment in itself helps to combat the demoralizing sense of isolation that typically accompanies illness. Two tangible symbols of both the physician's role and the world view supporting his treatment are medications and surgical operations, and the psychological effects of both may be striking. [59]

The psychological effects of medications and surgery can also be terrifying, and paradoxically hospitalization itself may be unfavorable to healing. A British study compared patients who were treated for coronary occlusion in an intensive-care unit with those who were treated at home. Results indicated that the atmosphere of emergency, crisis, and turmoil in the intensive-care unit can offset its technical advantages. Patients with comparable states of the disease who were treated at home lived longer.[57] Such studies employ the only measure that is easy to observe and document: the length of time a patient survives. The quality of life is difficult to assess, although many would say that it is more important than sheer survival time. In this case it would seem to tilt the balance of argument even more in favor of home care when that is possible.

However, such arguments can also be taken to support a fresh approach to the psychology of patient care in the hospital. The more psychiatric studies are carried out with hospitalized patients, the more convincing the argument becomes that the speed of healing can be influenced by enhancing or destroying the patient's confidence and expectation of recovery. Studies with patients undergoing surgery for detached retina, with servicemen being treated for infectious diseases, with children undergoing tonsillectomies, and with other surgical procedures bear this out.

Frank cites one simple but dramatic example: Forty-four children hospitalized for tonsillectomies were divided into two groups. One group had a ten-minute interview with a nurse, who explained the operation to them, told them what to expect and how they might feel after the surgery, and reassured them about the safety of the procedure. The other group received routine preoperative care. At the end of a week, the children who got the ten-minute interview had all been discharged from the hospital, while half of the other group were still hospitalized. The point is obvious, I think. If a patient is treated mechanistically, with a repair-shop atmosphere in the hospital, the likelihood of rapid, successful healing is less than if "expectant faith" is encouraged and fostered.

Relatively few studies have attempted to link the speed of recovery with the way a patient is dealt with personally, but those few provide confirmation for a major thesis of holistic medicine: Beliefs and emotions are as important in maintaining and recovering health as physiological measures are.

The Power of Placebos

The classic way to test a new medication is to administer it to half of an experimental group, administer an inert substance to the other half, and note the difference in the effects between the two groups. This is best done in a *double-blind* situation, where neither the subjects nor the people conducting the experiment know which group is receiving which substance. Any positive effect on the group receiving the inert substance is called the *placebo effect.*

In studies carried out since 1958, it has become clear that the placebo effect is something to be reckoned with. Studies of analgesics, for example, might be expected to reveal some relief from pain in those patients who believe that something is being done medically to alleviate their pain. In one study the inert placebo turned out to be 55 percent as effective as aspirin and, more surprisingly, 55 percent as effective as morphine.[66] Three other medications were tested, including one to lower blood pressure, and in each of those cases the percentage of relief obtained from the medically inert substance was in the neighborhood of 55 percent. In another study patients with bleeding peptic ulcers were injected with distilled water; they were told that this new medicine would cure them. In 70 percent of the cases the results were excellent, and they continued to be excellent during a full year's follow-up.[175] The interesting question here is what distinguishes the 55 percent, for whom the placebo works, from the others? And in the case of the patients with bleeding ulcers, what distinguishes the 70 percent, who recovered after the injections of distilled water, from those who didn't? What Sigmund Freud called "expectation colored by hope and faith" and what Jerome Frank calls "expectant faith" clearly are important. In the study with the peptic ulcer patients, another group was given the same injection of distilled water by a nurse who told them that it was an experimental procedure that might or might not help them. In that group only 25 percent showed remission of symptoms, as against the 70 percent who showed remission when told that it would cure them.

For generations physicians have been aware of the placebo effect, and many have deliberately dispensed mild or inert "medicines" to patients with insomnia or other ailments where the most important factor in the treatment seemed to be the patient's belief that something was being done, or where a symbol was needed of the physician's ability to cure the illness. Only recently has the placebo effect itself come under study. Jerome Frank and his colleagues have also carried out several studies of placebos with psychiatric patients, and the evidence is strong that the most important factor in most psychotherapy is the expectation of help.[57] Recent studies by Dr. Jon D. Levine at the University of California at San Francisco indicate that placebos may activate several of the system's natural responses that promote healing: endorphins, the internal pain-killers; steroids, which counteract inflammation; and the immune system itself, possibly by stimulating the production of interferon. Far from being fake medication for illusory symptoms, placebos and the placebo effect can and should be taken seriously as clues to new means to enhance the system's own ability to deal with pain and disease.

The placebo effect sometimes complicates attempts to assess the effectiveness of drugs. The sugar pill could legitimately be labeled "Proved effective in one-third of all cases and absolutely safe," as a current medical joke suggests, and it could be recommended on that basis not only for pain but also for inflammatory conditions such as arthritis and hay fever. Beyond that, recent studies by psychiatrist Arthur K. Shapiro at Manhattan's Mt. Sinai Medical Center and Dr. Herbert Benson at Boston's Beth Israel Hospital indicate that the attitude of patients and physicians toward drugs *and toward each other* can have a pronounced influence on the effectiveness of placebos. Benson finds that a physician's expressed enthusiasm about a medication can increase the placebo effect to about 80 percent, even though the medication proves to be medically "worthless." Conversely, he finds that an unsatisfactory doctor-patient relationship may account for unpleasant side effects such as nausea, pain, and dizziness when placebos are administered.[133]

Warts and other skin problems seem to be particularly responsive to placebos. If warts are painted with a brightly colored, medically inactive dye, and the patient is told that the warts will be gone when the dye finally wears away, the recovery rate is as good as it is with any other known treatment for warts.

It is difficult to say what part of any medical procedure consists of "active ingredients" and what part consists of an "inert placebo." The evidence is strong that pronounced and measurable physiological effects can be made to happen by the expectation that they will, and that in many cases such expectations are the most important factors in healing.

Faith Healing

Although faith healing is not within the scope of scientific medicine, the connections between belief that one has been helped and the measurable effects of surgical procedures and medications pose some interesting questions. It's easy to dismiss the claims of religious healers, especially if we don't share their religion. And it's easy to assume that any disease cured by the ministrations of a faith healer must be imaginary. But we can no longer defend such assumptions convincingly.

At present some careful work is being done concerning religious healing in primitive societies. Until recently most of the research was carried out by anthropologists and psychologists, while medical researchers largely dismissed anything that was bound up with religious beliefs (and therefore difficult to investigate scientifically). Now physicians are looking at "psychic surgeons," shamans, and faith healers, and several things are becoming clear. By all indications an element similar to psychotherapy is present in many of the healing practices carried out within a tribal community. The idiom in which the ailment is discussed by patient and healer may include detailed explanations of the disorder in terms of spirits or local deities, and the treatment often comes to its climax in a public ceremony that involves the entire community in an intense, emotional, cathartic ritual of exorcism, which leaves the patient exhausted, often feverish, and ultimately cured. A sharp distinction is rarely made in African societies, for example, between emotional illness and physical illness. Relief from what we would identify as severe depression can easily enough be understood in this framework. And even relief from the inflammation associated with gallstones and similar disorders, also reported, is not surprising in light of recent Western findings concerning the placebo effect. Where a patient is from a different community than the healer, two factors typically operate. The first is showmanship and skill, as exemplified by the famous "psychic surgeons" of the Philippines, who appear to remove portions of diseased tissue without the use of instruments, and in some cases without making an incision. By all indications, the intensity of emotion surrounding psychic surgery, coupled with the use of sleight-of-hand to produce a dramatic display of blood and tissue that seemingly comes from the patient, is designed to convince the patient that something drastic and decisive has been done.

The second factor is exemplified by the shrine at Lourdes. Here a worldwide institution gives support to the attitude of expectant faith. The preparation for the pilgrimage, the journey itself, the ceremonies and vigils at the shrine, all serve to reinforce the positive and expectant emotional attitude. Jerome Frank, who has studied the records of cures at Lourdes, notes that they are not instantaneous; they require time, but often less time than ordinary healing. "The processes by which cures at Lourdes occur do not seem to differ in kind from those involved in normal healing, although they are remarkably strengthened and accelerated."[57]

The holistic attempt to understand healing in terms of the entire human system rather than in terms of localized activities at the site of illness or injury, and to study the psychological aspects of healing in clinical situations, are significant steps beyond the fringe of what mechanistic medicine could study seriously. Psychic healing, ESP, psychokinesis, and such things as the laying on of hands constitute another fringe. Little hard evidence is available about them, and there is no unifying scheme by which to interpret the many anecdotal reports.[67] When we have a better understanding of the physiological effects of beliefs, expectations, attitudes, and long-range habits of emotion, and when these can be more clearly linked to the biochemistry of pain, inflammation, and immunity, it will be time for a closer look at the claims of psychics and faith healers.

Rational and Irrational Intervention

Traditionally, the use of hypnosis, persuasion, and placebos to manipulate a patient's beliefs have been regarded as "irrational" measures for the treatment of disease. There has always been a suspicion that symptoms relieved by such measures must have been illusory to begin with. From the emerging links among biochemistry, emotion, and healing, those suspicions are no longer well founded. Nevertheless, one can see why the largely conservative medical community wants to sort out "rational" procedures, such as surgical and chemical intervention, from "irrational" procedures. In the one case the causal connection between treatment and recovery is clear; in the other, it isn't, so far. But we are close to having rational explanations for the effectiveness of many "irrational" procedures.

One line of approach to such explanations involves complex biological responses that resemble the stress response and immune response. Both of these complicated biochemical activities are triggered in the hypothalamus by specific sorts of events in human experience. In the case of the stress response, the triggering is done by interpreted perceptions. Simonton's work with cancer patients and the results of some of the research with hypnosis, coupled with Jerome Frank's studies of accelerated rates of healing, suggest that the immune response can also be stimulated by perceptual cues. No doubt there are similar cases of physiological "responses" that can be initiated and manipulated by means other than chemical and surgical intervention.

What is called the "relaxation response" by researchers at Harvard Medical School is apparently controlled from the same area of the hypothalamus. It constitutes yet another set of complex biochemical activities, and it can be manipulated through specific and deliberate behavior. It wouldn't be at all surprising if the connection between the "arthritis-prone personality" discussed earlier and the onset of the disease was explained by showing that certain kinds of emotional habits are associated with the production of lower than normal amounts of the steroids that control inflammation. It is likely that the production of pain-killing endorphins and steroids, and even more subtle physiological activities, can be initiated by specific kinds of experience and deliberate behavior. All of this, as new as it is to the mainstream of medical research, must be understood as part of the natural biological capacity of the human organism to adapt to changing environmental conditions. The role of these aspects of our biological heritage in the recovery from disease and injury, and in the maintenance of health, is just beginning to come under serious and intense study.

The second line of explanation for the effectiveness of emotion and attitude in the treatment of clinical symptoms comes from recent advances in our understanding of the biochemistry of pain and emotion. In large measure, these advances have come about in the course of research into the effects of specific drugs. As "rational" as the use of drugs and medications seems to be on the basis of the strict clinical tests, there is often no explanation for *how* a specific drug acts to control anxiety, depression, or pain. Explanations have often been as elusive as explanations for the effectiveness of hypnosis and placebos. Once again, the block to a better understanding of such matters seems to be the traditional Western distinction between mind and body.

What you experience as moods and changes in emotional state *just are* changes in the biochemical characteristics of your system. The same events can be accurately described in either way. You might describe a given conscious activity by saying, "I raised my arm." A neurophysiologist might describe the activity by talking about neural events and muscular movement. There would be no doubt that you were both talking about the same event, but from two different points of view. In the same way, the conscious activities of thought, belief, and emotion are coincident with unconscious neurochemical activity. You *feel* those chemical changes, just as much as you feel a hot liquid in your mouth, and you have learned to describe those feelings in emotional terms.

The chemistry of mood and emotion is complicated, and the nature of unconscious chemical activity is just beginning to be untangled. But there is already enough information to provide at least a sketch of how "irrational" procedures may indeed be rational: The chemistry of emotion is linked to the chemistry of other natural activities, including the healing of wounds and the immune response on the positive side, and the generation of stress reactions and digestive problems on the negative side. To manipulate a person's experiences, beliefs, and emotions just is to manipulate the biochemical states.

A rational connection between emotional state and physiological state begins to emerge. Only one thing is involved: a whole, functioning person. What counts as *rational* intervention in the course of disease, now that we are beginning to understand these matters differently? In a clinical situation intervention is most effective when it involves manipulating the cognitive, emotional, and physiologica! states of the patient. That much of the argument in favor of holistic medicine is already clear. And to the extent that disease can now be understood in the context of a whole human life and the adaptation of a person to the conditions of his life, intervention in the course of disease will have to involve intervention in the course of day-to-day habits as well. Thus the responsibility must shift from the health professionals to the individual. The professionals can determine what is medically effective, they can intervene in emergencies, and they can provide medical and surgical treatment when it is appropriate. But they cannot determine our day-to-day habits, or the attitudes, reactions, and habits of emotional response that constitute an individual adjustment to the circumstances of an individual life. The responsibility of health professionals in these matters can only consist of education and counseling. It is likely that the primary role of the medical professional in most of our lives will shift over the next few years from that of a repairman to that of an adviser.

CHAPTER SIX

Holism and the Human Brain

Hypnosis is probably the prime recent example of the demystification of what were once considered to be inherently occult phenomena. Trance, despite its supernatural associations, is a natural event in human life. It happens spontaneously at times of deep relaxation or intense concentration, and it seems to provide an access for the conscious and deliberate regulation of ordinarily unconscious biological activity by manipulating the cues that trigger that activity.

Beliefs in ESP, psychokinesis, telepathy, clairvoyance, and psychic healing are ancient, and it is fair to ask why they have persisted. The gullibility of the general public isn't a convincing explanation. Legitimate questions can be asked, primarily about the existence of such events, and only secondarily about how they might be explained. But I don't see that the case for or against extrasensory phenomena is strengthened by the current research.

It is much too early in the game to start grinding the ESP axe on holistic medicine. There are perfectly ordinary biological events in human experience that need to be investigated first, and that investigation has just recently taken a significant turn toward establishing constructive connections among the many aspects of human experience. Solid, testable, scientific explanations are beginning to emerge for the connections that on the old Cartesian view had to be described as extending from the body to the mind on the one hand, and from the mind to the body on the other. On the holistic view, they are understood not in mind-body terms, but as relationships between different sorts of event that happen in the life of a person. Explaining them entails finding out more than we currently know about the workings of that least understood part of the human organism: the brain.

Exploring Neurochemistry

Every living organism has the ability to detect and to distinguish nourishment and danger, and to deal with them, if only to move toward the one and away from the other. In human beings, perhaps more than in other species, far more subtle discriminations are made. Unfortunately, there isn't yet a clear and well-differentiated vocabulary for describing and sorting out the physiological states that are linked to the ways we interpret situations. The technical vocabulary is even less clear when it comes to sorting out the interpretations themselves and the emotional contexts in which they occur. Such matters are vital if we are to understand our own biological responses.

The mugger who pulls a gun on you doesn't initiate the stress reaction. You first have to know what a gun is, to recognize it and the whole situation as constituting danger. We don't react to raw visual information; we have to interpret the information—categorize and assimilate it either consciously or unconsciously—before we *can* react to it at all. We know very little about how the brain, human or animal, interprets visual signals. Some interpretation may be innate and unlearned. Many psychological researchers think, for example, that most human beings have an innate reaction to visual forms that resemble snakes. But for the most part, interpretations are learned, although the connection between these learned perceptual responses and specific patterns of neural activity is not fully understood. On the other hand, we do know something of what happens *after* the cues are interpreted. The perceptual triggering of most physiological responses, by the best evidence now available, takes place in the hypothalamus, which secretes neural hormones that initiate specific biochemical activity in the pituitary, the adrenal cortex, and other organic systems, as well as in specific neural pathways in the brain and the spinal column.

When there is a disorder in the ways we interpret situations, or a disproportionate emotional and behavioral reaction to day-to-day experiences, we speak of mental illness, anxiety, neurosis, psychosis—conditions which have proved more difficult to deal with medically than most human disorders. Intervention in emotional disturbances, either by professionals or by the individual himself, has been complicated. Most of what we know about biochemical events in the human brain has been found out within the past twenty-five years, and new developments are occurring rapidly. However, people have been using chemical means to alter their own neurochemical states for thousands of years, for medical and other reasons. Alcohol, opiates, marijuana, and hallucinogens, for example, alter the character of chemical events in the brain and nervous system. Until twenty-five or thirty years ago, the usual medical means for intervening in severe states of anxiety or agitation were the barbiturates amytal and phenobarbitol, and while it wasn't known how they worked, it was clear that they were effective.

When the mood-altering drugs called tranquilizers were introduced during the 1950s, their dramatic effect on anxiety and psychosis was not well understood. Recent research has produced a clearer conception of what goes on in the brain during distinct states of emotional arousal and sensitivity to pain. Early research revealed that librium and valium have similar effects on virtually all species, from fish to chimpanzees. This suggests that the drugs act on a part of the brain that developed early in the evolutionary process, a part that we share with other species, and that the physiological activities involved are those which figure in very basic reactions to interpreted perceptual cues concerning danger. It is possible to study the effects of these drugs under a wider variety of experimental conditions than would have been feasible if the effects could be observed only in human subjects. In general, tranquilizers make a person or animal less concerned about danger and reduce fear of pain, frustration, punishment, disappointment, and of the consequences of actions. There is a decrease in anxiety, but no decrease in aggression. The drugs do not "tone down" the entire organism; they act selectively on specific activities in the brain.[68]

But the tranquilizers have many drawbacks. They are all toxic to some degree, especially if administered over a long period of time. And, in both human beings and experimental animals, they lessen the ability to notice change in the environment and to respond to new events. Anyone who has had to drive a car after one drink too many is familiar with this effect of alcohol, and many people experience the same effect with tranquilizers. Finally, these drugs make one less likely to persist toward goals when the environment is unpredictable. Neither animals nor people toughen up and adapt to change and adversity when they are tranquilized.[178] But as means for medical intervention in severe psychiatric disorders, tranquilizers and related drugs have revolutionized the treatment of mental illness, making it possible for the number of patients confined in mental hospitals to be reduced drastically, from more than a half-million in 1956 to fewer than 200,000 at present.[18] However, critics suggest that alleviating severe symptoms by means of tranquilizers puts off coping with underlying problems, and that many of the patients released are simply not ready to deal with the world outside the mental hospitals, even with the aid of medication. As with any dramatic new therapy, it is possible that the tranquilizers have been overused and that their effectiveness in bringing about permanent remission of symptoms has been overestimated.

Neurotransmitters and Neuromodulators

The effects of the psychoactive drugs opened up a series of questions about how emotional states are related to physiological processes. Recently, answers have begun to accumulate rapidly. Substances that are known to affect brain function can be traced through the system by scanning devices. The use of the electron microscope to identify specific characteristics of neural cells, and in some cases to examine chemical structures down to the molecular level, has not only increased the rate of discovery, but has connected data from a variety of sources.

It is tempting and convenient to think of the human brain as a great computer, but it is misleading too, even though some human problem-solving activities can be imitated at dazzling speed by digital computers. The brain and the nervous system are not composed of a fixed set of cells processing information electrically or electronically, as was thought to be the case in the 1950s. Rather, complex chemical directors in the brain and throughout the nervous system influence how information will be handled and in some cases bear information themselves. Coming to understand them has given researchers a new picture of how the brain works.

The brain consists of more than 15 billion neurons that are connected in complex patterns. Specific areas of the brain are associated with particular functions. Portions of the cortex are connected with the movement of specific parts of the body; other portions with sensation, speech, problem-solving, and visualization. The limbic system, a doughnut-shaped area deep inside the brain, is identified with a broad range of emotional activities. Other specific areas are associated with the transmission of signals of chronic pain, and still others with those of transient, acute pain.

Neurons aren't "wired together," as the electrical conception of the brain that was common thirty years ago would suggest. There is a small gap between adjacent neurons, called the *synapse,* or synaptic cleft. The connection across this gap is made by a *neurotransmitter,* a chemical that is released by one neuron and diffuses across the gap to trigger specific electrochemical activity in the next. The transmitters interact with receptors in the "receiving" neurons in a lock-and-key arrangement governed by the actual shape of the molecules of the transmitter. This shape and fit is important: Many psychoactive drugs affecting mood and sensitivity to pain are effective because they resemble specific neurotransmitters; they fool receptor sites on neural cells into accepting them instead of the brain's own chemical transmitters, either facilitating or inhibiting the natural rate of transmission. When the signal between two neurons has passed, the neurotransmitter is either destroyed by the metabolic processes of the brain and bloodstream, or it is removed from the cleft in a "reuptake" phase, in which it is transferred from the synaptic cleft back to the first of the two neurons, then stored for re-use or broken down by enzymes. In the average brain, there are about 100,000 such chemical reactions every second.

The monamines seem to be the most important neuro-transmitters: dopamine, serotonin, epinephrine, and norepi-nephrine. Dopamine and norepinephrine in particular domi-nate the action in the nerve pathways in the brain that are most prominent in transmitting the signals of perceptions and emo-tions. During the 1960s research into the chemical treatment of schizophrenia concentrated on two facts: Specific tran-quilizers, in particular chlorpromazine, seemed to correct the thought disorders and lessen hallucinations; and an overdose of amphetamines produced symptoms of a drug psychosis remarkably similar to the symptoms of schizophrenia.

These findings illustrate the chain of discovery that takes form rapidly when a new sort of scientific question emerges. A race began among researchers already working on a number of related questions about the chemical basis of drug addiciton, the pathways of pain impulses in the nervous system, the neurochemical activities involved in perception, memory and learning. All of them zeroed in on untangling the complicated chemical activity that passes impulses from one neuron to another in the brain, the spinal column, and throughout the nervous system. It became apparent that the tranquilizers inhibited the release of the neurotransmitter dopamine from its tiny storage areas in specific brain cells, thus tuning down the emotional and perceptual action along specific neural path-ways. The amphetamines, on the other hand, speeded and intensified the action by causing the release of an excess of norepinephrine, while at the same time arresting the "limiting" action that normally keeps the amount of this transmitter at any neural junction in proportion. The result is the jangling "high," that just is the experience of greatly accelerated neural messages across the synapses governed by norepinephrine.

The hypothesis emerged rather quickly that schizophrenia could be identified with irregularities in the production and release of these two neurotransmitters. Chlorpromazine became the first line of attack on schizophrenia, and it was successful in a large percentage of cases. But it also failed in many cases. Just when the researchers thought there were only a few more details to be worked out, a whole new area of inquiry opened up.

It began to appear that the action of the tranquilizers in inhibiting dopamine release amounted to tinkering with a chain of disordered brain processes somewhere in the middle; that the basic chemical disorder that lay at the root of schizophrenia was somewhere earlier along in the chain of events. Further questions had to be investigated: about the nature of the receptor sites on neurons, and about other substances within the neurons that facilitated the transfer of signals from the receptors to the interior of the cells. It became clear that not all of the receptors were "locks" into which the "keys" of neurotransmitters fitted. Other substances were involved which adjusted and tempered the transmission of signals, and there were specific neural locks for which *they* were the keys. These substances were identified as enzymes and other proteins, some of them peptide hormones generated in the pituitary gland and directly associated with the fight-or-flight response.

Pieces of the puzzle fell together rapidly, integrating research on other aspects of brain activity with the new information about the chemical character of synaptic events. The roles of specific neurotransmitters in particular areas of the brain began to come clear. A review of the research reports published up to the middle of 1978 lists forty-one different chemicals and groups of chemicals that regulate neural activity.[14] In addition to the neurotransmitters, a large class of chemicals, now called *neuromodulators*, alter in one way or another the characteristics of the signals conveyed by the neurotransmitters. As their role has become apparent, the distinction between mind and matter has become something more than a conceptual inconvenience; it has become scientifically untenable.

Neuromodulators affect the activity along pathways in the brain and the spinal column by bonding to specialized receptors on the neurons in those pathways. The sites are "coded," so that only molecules of certain shapes can bond to them. In 1973 Candace Pert at Johns Hopkins, working with Dr. Solomon Snyder, found that receptor sites in specific regions of the brain are associated with transmitting signals of chronic pain. These sites accept the molecules of the opiates morphine and heroin. The network of opiate receptor sites also coincides closely with the neural pathways of perception and emotion.

Why are certain sites in the brain seemingly designed to receive chemicals such as opium? The answer could only be that there were substances in the brain itself that resembled opium and figured in the human system's own modulation of pain, perception, and emotion. By 1975 the chemicals were found. Called *endorphins,* the internal morphines, they are peptide hormones, produced in several forms in the brain and the pituitary gland. They act in precisely the same way as morphine and heroin, modulating pain signals and at the same time affecting the transmission of perceptual and emotional signals. But the endorphins are 30 to 100 times more powerful than morphine in relieving pain.

The psychoactive drugs, then, mimic substances that are naturally present in the brain and nervous system, and that act on particular functions because the neurons that have receptor sites to accept the chemicals are concentrated in the areas of the brain and nervous system which are specialized pathways for particular kinds of signal.

Under certain circumstances people who have been severely injured can keep right on functioning for a time, seemingly oblivious to pain. In certain states of concentration or religious ecstasy people can walk on hot coals. The pain of childbirth can be diminished by training sessions in natural childbirth. Why? The hypothesis is that the natural production of endorphins in the human system can be increased by specific kinds of stimulation. We make our *own* morphine, right in our brains.

Many neuroscientists suspect that people who are susceptible to drug addiction have a deficiency in natural endorphins. The discovery of endorphins, and particularly the group called *enkephalins*, which modulate the activity along the pathways associated with sensation and many emotional reactions, opens a new chapter in the study of pain, drug addiction, and psychiatric disorders.

What is startling about the neuromodulators, as they appear one by one, is that their action is so specific. Again, animal research has shown that some neuromodulators affect learning and memory: When the modulators are present, learning is rapid; when they are absent, it doesn't happen at all. Some psychoactive drugs—amphetamines, mescaline, psilocon, LSD, and DMT—can induce psychosis since they closely resemble the natural neuromodulators in the brain. A greater understanding of their function should therefore provide specific ways to deal with psychoses. New drug therapies are in the offing.

But drugs, artificially produced neurochemicals, tranquilizers, and other psychoactive substances, with their toxic side effects, may not be the most desirable ways of dealing with problems of chemical imbalance in the brain. It has come as a surprise to many medical people in the past few years that the activity of specific brain neurons varies in response to normal fluctuations in the diet.[90] *Precursors*, substances which the system uses to manufacture the neurotransmitters, are contained in the foods we eat. The rate at which the brain synthesizes the neurotransmitters changes in proportion to the amounts of the precursors in the diet and in the bloodstream.

One of the neurotransmitters that has been manipulated in clinical situations by dietary means is *acetylcholine*. Deficiencies in this substance can produce *tardive dyskenesia,* a disfiguring condition involving involuntary twitches of the facial muscles. Working on the hypothesis that deficiencies in acetylcholine can be corrected by increasing the amount of its precursor *choline* in the diet, psychiatrists at Stanford, Tufts, the University of Montreal, and other universities have begun feeding patients lecithin, a choline-rich derivative of soybeans that is used in the food industry as an emulsifier. The results, reported at a meeting in Tucson in December 1978, were uniformly successful. Lecithin also shows promise in the treatment of mania and senile dementia, which may also be connected with deficiencies in acetylcholine. There is enough encouraging evidence to suggest that the "precursor" approach to manipulating neural chemistry by altering a patient's diet will be effective in other disorders as well. In experiments carried out in Sweden, increasing dietary amounts of amino acids, which are precursors of the neurotransmitters in the catecholamine group, shows promise as a treatment for depression.[90]

One of the amino acids essential in the human diet, *tryptophan,* is a precursor of the neurotransmitter serotonin. Low levels of serotonin in the system are associated with depression and insomnia. In a number of clinical studies in this country and England, large doses of tryptophan and niacinamide (vitamin B3) were given to depressed patients, with positive results. In one British study, patients receiving the precursor nutrients were compared with a group who were receiving twice-weekly electroconvulsive shock treatments, a standard treatment for severe depression. Beginning about the tenth day and extending through the following weeks of the study, the patients who received tryptophan showed more positive results than those receiving shock therapy.[103] Similar comparison studies have shown the use of tryptophan and niacinamide to be as effective as well-known antidepressant drugs like imipramine,[135] and trials at Boston State Hospital have shown the treatment to be effective for insomnia as well.[72] Increasing the intake of the mineral lithium over a long period prevents the development of supersensitivity of neural receptors for the neurotransmitter dopamine. Its effectiveness in preventing recurrent manic-depressive episodes is well established.[127]

Such measures, which involve either changes in long-range dietary habit or temporary supplementation with high pharmacological doses of specific nutritional substances, suggest that the prevention and in some cases the treatment of emotional disorders may be approached through changes in personal habit over a period of time rather than by the more dramatic and sometimes jarring direct intervention in the chemistry of the brain and nervous system.

Biochemical Habits and Responses

The central nervous system, understood as an organ of the human system, is more complex than all the other organs put together. Its characteristics and functions are constantly changing in response to events in the environment, to specific physiological states of arousal or relaxation, to states of disease within the overall system, and as the result of the natural course of human experience. Many chemical characteristics of your nervous system were acquired—learned—over the course of your life until now. They have been shaped by your experiences.

Suppose, for example, that a child grows up in a situation where there are constant emergencies in the household, constant changes in his living situation with no prior warning or preparation, constant threats to his well-being, and frequent emotional turmoil. He learns, after a time, to be prepared—primed to cope with emergency at every moment. The expectation is "trained in"; It becomes a pattern of habit to be always on guard, and the pattern is reflected in habitual biochemical states as the child matures. The individual's normal levels of specific neurochemicals will be quite different from those of a person who grew up in a situation where he knew pretty well what to expect from one day to the next.

Normal levels and a normal balance and proportion of the neurotransmitters and modulators, differ from one person to another according to habituation, nutrition, and genetic makeup. To some extent emotional characteristics and tendencies are inherited, no doubt because of inherited differences in the natural biochemical balance of neuroregulatory processes. Nasty tempers do, literally, run in families, and some animal studies have shown that certain forms of aggression are clearly inherited.[14] But more subtle patterns of emotional response must also be affected by inherited biochemical characteristics.

At the same time, experience forms, strengthens and reinforces biochemical habits, affecting a person's normal levels of activity in places other than the brain. For example, a person who ate only raw foods for some years—fruits, vegetables, nuts—would have a different set of chemical "expectations" in his digestive system than one whose diet consisted only of bland, overcooked foods. The "raw foods" person getting ready to sit down to a meal, would be preparing himself chemically for a different kind of digestive activity than the "overcooked" person would, even before the food is consumed. In fact, the "overcooked" person would have trouble digesting the other's diet, and vice versa. But over a period of time, either one could probably *learn* to accommodate the other diet. Thus, deliberately repeated behavior and carefully cultivated habits can change unconscious biochemical habits. And that "training" can take place in the brain as well as in the digestive system.

Within the limits set by inherited characteristics, the kinds of experience we have influence the setting of what have been called *regulostats*. These establish the particular "resting" rate of neural activity, the normal range of reaction to specific kinds of perceived situations, and the relative "mix" of different kinds of neural signals, determining which are likely to be stronger, which slower or faster, and so on.[14] Once again, extreme cases can illuminate ordinary ones. Mental illness can now be understood in terms of neurochemicals. In susceptible individuals, repeated experience of extreme psychological states can alter the activity of the neuroregulators to such a degree that behavior in stressful situations becomes pathological.

This new understanding of mental illness suggests an approach to the development of new pharmacological treatments, following the direction set by the use of tranquilizers. But perhaps more interesting, it suggests the development of improved *environmental* treatments. A mentally disturbed person's "base-line" level of neural activity might be manipulated by changing the character of his experience. Over a period of time, a new base-line is established. The unconscious neurochemical activity is litterally retrained.

Holism and Brain Chemistry

Long-term habits of emotion and behavior affect the biochemical states of the brain and vice versa, in a mutually supporting relationship: the more a behavior is repeated, the more the neurochemical situation is modified to make it likely that it will be repeated again. In addition to therapeutic "retraining," biochemical states can be altered in specific ways by introducing small amounts of the chemical neuroregulators or their precursors into the system, or by using psychoactive drugs. The connections between diet and brain chemistry suggest even more possibilities for both the occasional intervention and the long-range alteration of patterns of emotion and behavior.

Beyond this, there are situations in which specific neuroregulators are released in unusual amounts, as in the case of severe injury. Some situational stimuli cause the release of peptide hormones which affect neural activity in such a way as to facilitate learning and memory, or to initiate or suppress the stress response and other complex hormonal activities.[14]

Now comes a particularly holistic question: Can we learn to *manipulate* our own perceptions and behavior so as to influence our physiological and behavioral states without chemicals? Can we learn to tranquilize ourselves at will, to control pain by triggering our own internal opiates, to stimulate our immune systems? The answer may very well be *yes,* but the clues as to how such natural and ordinarily unconscious processes can be manipulated are just beginning to appear. There is good reason to believe that the use of hypnosis in the control of chronic pain triggers the release in the brain of the "internal opiate" beta-endorphin.[61] Evidence is beginning to accumulate that activities such as jogging, when carried on for a sufficient time, can trigger the release of some of the peptide neuromodulators that inhibit depression and promote emotional stability. Hypnosis, meditation, intense concentration, and other voluntary "altered states of consciousness" can change the amounts and proportions of neurochemicals in the brain and the nervous system.

From a biological point of view, the principal function of the brain is to transform sensory events into appropriate activities, both conscious and unconscious. Altered states of consciousness promise to provide access to the complex chemical activities of the brain and nervous system by allowing us to alter the perceptions that ordinarily initiate such activities. Remember that we share many of the biological responses with other species. The fight-or-flight response, for example, exists on a primitive level of consciousness, uninvolved with complex conceptual and linguistic activity. That would explain why, in the use of hypnosis for pain control, visual imagery has proven to be more effective than the direct verbal instruction to feel less pain: the imagery takes the place of the *perceptual* cues that naturally trigger the release of appropriate biochemicals. It also gives a clue to the effectiveness of visual imagery in Simonton's work with cancer patients. In addition, the extraordinary feats of physical control and analgesia that are practiced in the mystical traditions of other cultures become more comprehensible in this light. Alien medical and psychological procedures that we were once ready to dismiss because they "can't work" are beginning to gain serious respect.

There is a line of connection to be sketched at present and filled out in more detail by future research, between what we have traditionally identified as mental activities and physical activities. It is a complicated but perfectly straightforward line of scientific, testable, rational explanation of the relationships among different kinds of event in the life of a person. It is clear that we can come to understand, alter, and take responsibility for conditions in our lives that we once thought were far beyond our control.

CHAPTER SEVEN

Other People's Medicine

The Appeal of Alien Idioms

If all the biological responses we've been talking about are a part of human nature and have been for tens of thousands of years, then why haven't we learned to control them to our advantage before this? We have, if you let the "we" cover the whole human race. Many of the practices of non-Western medicine exploit precisely those biological responses and activities that have been getting so much attention recently in Western medicine and psychology. In large measure they do so by altering individual experience rather than by manipulating physiological states chemically or surgically.

I don't mean to suggest, of course, that non-Western science has understood the role of the hypothalamus and the pituitary, or the chemical neurotransmitters and neuroregulators, any more than we have. But the functional and essentially organic understanding of both human beings and nature that characterizes Eastern thought constitutes an idiom of science that asks different questions about human health and well-being than have been asked in the West, and gets different answers.

Make no mistake about it, there is a solid scientific tradition in the East, and there has been for as long as there has been one in the West. To say that Oriental medical science isn't really science is like saying that Oriental music isn't really music. Its harmonies may be unfamiliar, but try to set down a decent definition of the term "music" that excludes it and you're going to end up trapped in your own particular tastes.

A society, as Robert Ardrey says, is a group of varied and unequal human beings organized to meet common needs. Part of what is involved in meeting needs is figuring out *how* to meet them and that, in large measure, is determined by matters of style and local idiom. A successful solution to one problem influences the approach to the next one, and a traditional way of developing solutions to problems becomes established.

The sciences in Eastern cultures typically begin with psychology, whereas the Western sciences have clustered around physics. Until recently, Western medicine has not understood the basic premises and intent of the Eastern psychologies. There has been little respect and some antagonism between the two traditions. The technology of Western physical science has made it possible for us to prosper, while Eastern cultures have been largely unable to feed and clothe their growing populations. However, we have not learned to engage our own wills to control our scientific achievements, or even to manage our individual lives very well. We have typically not seen ourselves as a part of nature.

There has been growing discontent within Western society about the extent to which technological advances are used without regard for human well-being or the environment, and about the depersonalization that results from a mechanistic approach to medicine and health. Perhaps the most striking evidence of discontent has been the enormous interest that has developed in Eastern philosophy and the disciplines of Zen, yoga, and other forms of meditation, as well as the willingness of many people to experiment with acupuncture and other medical procedures that are alien to the Western tradition of science. In many cases people have felt confronted with a choice between two cultures: either you accept the mechanistic view of the West, or you accept the mystical view of the East.[118]

Alternatively, interest has grown in the culture of American Indians—the native Americans. A good part of that renewed interest can be attributed to what they represent to us: a people who, before European colonization, lived a life that was openly based on an acceptance of the connection between man and nature. This is precisely the orientation that was missing during the rapid rise of mechanistic science in the West, and it has come to symbolize the closer integration of oneself with one's surroundings that is a part of the holistic movement.

In the industrialized West, healing is typically considered to be a private matter between patient and physician. In more homogeneous, tightly knit communities, among native Americans, Africans, and rural Orientals, healing has traditionally been an integral part of the social and religious life of the entire community.

Among the Navajos in Arizona and New Mexico, there is a unique blend of modern medicine and traditional healing. They may go to a modern hospital for surgery, but an important part of the recuperation from surgery, apparently a requisite for "feeling well" again, consists of having the community medicine man chant one of the traditional ceremonies for the patient. The ceremony serves the important and legitimate purpose of restoring patients to their own society and culture, and it depends upon the existence of shared beliefs and a tightly knit, personal orientation toward one's community to mark the transition from sickness to health.[140] Consistent with Jerome Frank's observations of the effects of "expectant faith" on the speed with which people recover from surgery, there seems to be a clear connection between the patient's belief that something has been done for the illness in a way that is understood by both the patient and those around him, and the rate, nature, and permanence of the recovery.

No one would suggest, of course, that a Navajo chant would be appropriate to mark the return of a patient to the home community in Scarsdale after gall bladder surgery. Modern urban society has no ceremony to mark the transition from sickness to health; it has no specific set of shared beliefs and symbols that have a psychological impact on all the members of a community to signify that the patient is supposed to be well now, and is expected to be. For the Navajos, having the entire neighborhood witness the medicine man perform the chant called "Blessing Way" signifies precisely that. The closest thing most of us have to a "getting well" ceremony is the inevitable stop at the cashier's window as we leave the hospital. It just doesn't do the job.

Among the Yoruba people in Africa, a similar sense exists of the connection between an individual's health and his place in the community. Health and disease are understood as indicators of the degree to which a person lives in peace and harmony within the community, and within the religious and tribal laws. Healing is a part of the society and the religion, and it involves the entire community. Sick people consult diviners and healers in order to find out the nature of their illness. The diagnosis and explanation are couched in the idioms and symbols of the local nature religion. In some cases, especially in what a Western scientist would diagnose as an emotional problem, treatment consists of a prolonged public ceremony, generating a dramatic psychological crisis in the patient, followed by a ceremonial reconciliation with the community. Even when preparations of known medicinal value are used, their administration is accompanied by ritual and ceremony, and their effectiveness is understood within the symbolic context of community beliefs.[95]

The question isn't whether or not such symbolic healings can be as effective as modern Western medicine in dealing with severe infectious illnesses and injuries. In most cases, of course, they cannot. The question is whether or not they are effective at all, for any type of disorder, and what role the shared beliefs play in the healing process.

Symptoms, Disease, and Diagnosis

The notion that a scientific tradition constitutes a *school of thought* should be taken more seriously than it generally is. Whether the subject matter is medicine or physics, chemistry or biology, there is clearly, at any time and place in human intellectual history, a clear-cut teaching function of a scientific community that prepares individuals to fill the vacancies left as older professionals retire or die. What is preserved and passed along is not only a set of techniques and the orthodox explanations for their effectiveness, but a point of view that determines what is and what is not acceptable in theory and practice, and what constitutes a "rational" approach to solving common problems.[157]

A view of nature will persist only to the extent that it yields effective ways of dealing with problems of human life. In China, in particular, there is a long tradition of science and technology that paralleled that of the West until about the seventeenth century. To some extent technological developments were exchanged between East and West. Many of the inventions that aided the rapid advance of European civilization originated in the East: printing, gunpowder, the compass, the seismograph, mechanical clockwork, segmental arch bridges, and, perhaps most important of all in doing the work of a growing civilization, stirrups and the horse collar. The view of the world that led to these successes differed from the Western view, but it got results.

The key to the Chinese understanding of nature is the concept of energy, *ch'i,* which is analogous to the current Western concept of a *field* of energy. The presence of matter in individual objects and in the human body is understood by the Chinese to be a rhythmic condensation of the energy that permeates the entire universe. Changes in the state of the energy are interpreted in terms of the concepts *yang* and *yin,* and in terms of five elements: metal, earth, wood, fire, and water. The energy in the human body is described in terms of fullness and emptiness, exteriority and interiority, cold and hot. The medical technique known as *acupuncture* is understood to modify the flow of the energy that constitutes the human system.

The most interesting part of traditional Chinese medicine is not acupuncture itself, but the detailed diagnostic procedures that precede its use. If the human system is viewed as an organized field of energy, with specific bodily structures seen as parts of the overall field, then diagnostic questions will pertain to the flow of energy into and around specific organs. In illness, how is the flow of energy disrupted? Sometimes the disruptions will be sought at places other than where symptoms appear.

When you put a rock or a stick into a flowing stream of water, it causes turbulence somewhere downstream, perhaps originating from the obstruction in an obvious way and perhaps not. If you want to end the turbulence, you don't try to push the surface of the water back into shape by brute force. You trace the flow back to the obstruction and remove it. When the human system is understood in this way, measures that seem reasonable for dealing with illness will be quite different from those taken on a mechanistic understanding. A toothache might be treated by stimulating or impeding the flow of energy at a point in the *hand* rather than in the tooth, and the appropriate place to manipulate the flow of energy in order to correct heart symptoms might well be in the feet.

The development of effective therapeutic techniques required evidence of the patterns of the flow of energy through the system. This is something different from the flow of blood and other fluids, which are taken to be condensations of that energy, just as tissues are. A pattern of evidence emerged from experiment that stood up to further testing and criticism: when a given function of the system is impaired, or a given organ is painful or malfunctions, certain areas of the skin become sensitive to the touch. From one individual to the next, the sensitive areas of the skin associated with specific diseases are about the same, and they are distributed along the surface of the body at some distance from the area where symptoms manifest themselves. This was understood to be evidence of the pathways along which the energy flowed through the body. The next step was to chart the flow of energy by tracing the points of sensitivity associated with specific diseases and organic systems. What emerged is the familiar acupuncture chart of the human body, which shows lines of connection between the points, *meridians,* or channels along which the *ch'i* force is understood to flow. Each meridian is identified with the major organ or function associated with it. The meridian associated with the lungs, for example, extends from the upper chest down through the arms to the thumb, with specific points identified where the energy flow is accessible to manipulation.

One question that has bothered Western scientists is whether the points defining the meridians have any characteristics that can be detected and measured. Aside from the sensitivity of the points during illness, which provided the original data for charting them, at least two characteristics have been found in the course of contemporary research in Japan. The electrical resistance of the skin drops appreciably at the points indicated by the acupuncture chart. Moreover, the meridians that connect the points exhibit distinct patterns of electrical permeability under specific conditions. Patients who have whiplash injuries, for example, were found to have a particular pattern of aberrant electrical activity along the traditional meridians, and this was consistent in the examination of more than a thousand cases.[105]

The diagnosis of a patient's disorder begins, like a Western diagnosis, with an interview to determine the patient's symptoms, the history of the trouble, the intensity, location and duration of any pain, and something of the patient's life, habits, and family history. From the beginning of the diagnostic session, the practitioner organizes information in terms of the twelve meridians and the five elements. This idiomatic technique of diagnosis dates back to the third century B.C., and it includes a prescribed set of "simple questions" that reflect philosophical concepts used in the classification of signs and symptoms and ultimately in the choice and administration of therapy.

Dr. Peter Rubin, a physician at Thomas Jefferson University School of Medicine, has been trained in traditional acupuncture as well as in Western medicine. The Oriental diagnostic system is so useful that Rubin says it is difficult to tell whether he uses Eastern or Western diagnosis more in his practice. Gathering of information is formalized and divided into inspection by each of the senses: observation of the tongue and the face as well as the posture and gait, interrogation for the tone of voice as well as for the answers to specific questions, listening to the sounds of the body, characteristic smells, and palpation of the radial and carotid pulses, the abdomen, and the texture of the skin.[2]

Observed characteristics come in groups of five, associated with the five Oriental elements. The conceptual scheme for organizing the diagnostician's perceptions of the sound of a patient's voice, for example, include a weeping quality or sadness associated with *metal,* a singing quality associated with *earth*, shouting or the lack of it associated with *wood*, laughter or the lack of it associated with *fire*, and a groaning quality associated with *water*. According to Rubin, the scheme is effective in organizing his impressions of a patient into a useful picture of the overall problem. If a patient has an imbalance of the element fire, Rubin says, there really is a lack of fire; the smile is empty. A "wooden" quality to the walk tends to correspond to a "wooden" quality in the voice.

Detecting disorders through odors is strange to Western medicine because it has no classificatory scheme for organizing and describing them. But curiously enough, Western researchers working with the symptoms of specific vitamin and mineral deficiencies often develop a "knack" after a time for picking out those patients who are deficient in certain nutrients by means of odor. Dr. Jonathan V. Wright, who has done research on the need for magnesium in human nutrition, says that a particular bodily smell associated with magnesium deficiency can be identified. But in modern Western medicine, research money isn't easily available for the study of odor as a means of diagnosis.

The Chinese scheme for classifying symptoms, disorders, and treatments can't be said either to succeed or to fail in describing the human system as it "really is." There are as many different idioms for describing the conditions of the human system accurately as there are for describing anything else. The test of a diagnostic scheme is whether or not it provides ways of detecting disorders in the system and leads to effective treatment. And the Chinese approach seems to do that. Modern studies carried out in China and in the West since 1955 have shown that many of the differentiations between normal and abnormal states made by the traditional diagnostic system correspond to measurable states that can be detected by modern means. For example, patients who were diagnosed by traditional means as having "kidney-sphere emptiness" were divided into groups that either had combined "yin and yang emptiness" or simply "yang emptiness." The differentiation corresponded to measurements of cortisone metabolites in the patients' urine, indicating that "the traditional diagnostic system could differentiate between hyper- and hypo-function of the adrenal cortex."[2]

Some specific therapeutic measures, "irrational" in Western terms, but rational as they can be in traditional Chinese terms, have proven to be successful in cases where modern therapy yields only partial results. In the past decade the traditional acupuncture techniques for producing anesthesia have been tried on laboratory animals, and electroencephalogram measurements have shown that stimulation in one area of the body can indeed produce measurable effects in distant areas that lie along an acupuncture meridian.

Many Western health professionals feel that we can learn from traditional Chinese medicine in the area where it has been most successful: the early detection of disease. Because traditional Oriental medicine could not deal effectively with severe organic and structural damage, it regarded this state of disease as advanced, or terminal, the result of either the patient's negligence or the physician's incompetence. It set about to find means of diagnosing and treating illness at an earlier stage.

The functioning of the human system is often disrupted long before recognizable organic damage takes place. Such serious organic diseases as cardiac failure, diabetes, and many forms of cancer are preceded by stages of progressive disorder in function. Western medicine usually does not detect disease at this stage or offer specific treatment, whereas Chinese medicine is often able to differentiate functional symptoms and offer specific therapy before there is structural damage.[131] The radical therapeutic techniques of modern medicine are scientific triumphs, but the aim of preserving health must be to detect and deal with disorders before such radical measures become necessary.

In Oriental medicine a specific complaint is regarded as only a symptom of a more general disorder. Where a Western physician diagnoses a duodenal ulcer, for example, the Chinese physician would understand the ulcer as a symptom. The ailment diagnosed is more likely to be an overall imbalance of the system. J. R. Worsley, who has been a professor of acupuncture in both China and Great Britain, writes:

> The traditional Chinese doctor looks upon all complaints as symptoms of trouble in the body, as manifestations of disease. He is trained to treat the cause, not the disorder, and tries to restore the life force to the parts of the body in which it was deficient so that the whole body is brought once again into balance. The disorder will then disappear of itself.[185]

The life force, ch'i, permeates the body on the Chinese understanding. Its balance is restored by stimulating specific points along the meridians by means of very fine needles, heat, massage, or the burning of a substance called moxa (wormwood) on or near the skin.

Acupuncture: The Fad and the Facts

During the initial enthusiasm which accompanied the recent rediscovery of acupuncture by the Western public, many excessive claims were made. Acupuncture became a medical fad for a time, and many believed that it offered a miracle cure for advanced diseases of the sort that no Eastern practitioner would approach with the technique. Some critics of Western medical philosophy seized upon acupuncture as the final refutation of mechanistic medicine. Of course, acupuncture is not a miracle cure. In the advanced stages of disease it has little to offer except relief from pain.

In China and Japan acupuncture is used alongside modern medicine to relieve certain ills and discomforts. The traditional means of diagnosis and treatment are effective in three principal ways: sedation, including the relief of pain; relaxation of tension and the overactivity of specific organ systems; and the modification of specific organic functions, including the regulation of excessive bleeding, depression, constipation or diarrhea, menstrual disorders, and problems of sexual function. The complaints for which it is most effective are those which occur at the early stages of disease: headache, cramps, muscular pain, referred pain, neuralgia, and the first phases of inflammatory disorders such as arthritis.[105]

There has been a good deal of speculation that acupuncture is effective largely because of the placebo effect. To some extent this is true of any medical technique, but acupuncture is used successfully in veterinary medicine as well as in human medicine, which suggests that there is a good deal more to it than that.

Most of us heard about acupuncture for the first time within the past decade. Actually, it has been known in the West for about 300 years. A Dutch physician, Willem Ten Rhijne, worked for the Dutch East India Company in Nagasaki from 1674 to 1676, and he learned about traditional Oriental medicine in his travels across India, China, and Japan. When he returned to the Netherlands, he used acupuncture in treating his patients, and in 1683 he wrote a book explaining the technique and introducing the term acupuncture, which he put together from two Latin roots. At about the same time, a German physician, also in Nagasaki, brought the technique back to Leyden. By 1821 acupuncture was being used in France and England, and in 1825 an article on the subject was translated from the French and published in Philadelphia by Benjamin Franklin's grandson, Dr. Franklin Bache. Bache became well known for his research on acupuncture with twelve prisoners at the state prison in Philadelphia, where he was the assistant physician. As far as is known, the treatment was never used outside Philadelphia.

This was before Louis Pasteur's work, which led to an understanding of germs and the need for sterilization, and infection came to be a serious problem in the use of acupuncture. The technique was not generally accepted, despite a second revival of interest late in the nineteenth century with the work of Sir William Osler, a Canadian physician.

There is little doubt that acupuncture helps many patients, especially if it is used at the early stage of illness, the way it is in Oriental societies. The relief of certain symptoms is fairly reliable, but there is no way to tell whether the symptoms relieved *would have* turned into a serious organic disease without the treatment. The advocates of acupuncture will of course believe that such is the case, while the skeptics will not.

The one area where acupuncture's effectiveness has been accepted by much of the Western medical community is in the relief of pain. Several different explanations have been offered for the success of the technique. Ronald Melzack, in *The Puzzle of Pain,* advances the hypothesis that two major kinds of nerve fiber are involved in the transmission of pain: large *A-beta* fibers, which respond to nonpainful stimuli, and smaller *c-fibers,* which respond to painful stimuli. If the activity of the larger fibers is increased, Melzack suggests that a spinal "gate" is closed, inhibiting the transmission of pain signals along the c-fibers. He suggests that acupuncture needles selectively stimulate the larger fibers, and the increased activity closes the "gate," thus inhibiting the transmission of pain signals.[113] Extending Melzack's hypothesis, other clinical researchers have postulated that there is a second gate located higher in the nervous system, which would account for the alleviation of head pain.

It seems likely that the gate theory will be absorbed by the recent work on endorphins. The gates may be areas where there are high concentrations of endorphin receptors, or perhaps junctions of neural pathways that have the receptors. Studies by B. Sjölund in Sweden and Chang Hsiang-tung in Shanghai indicate that acupuncture triggers the liberation in the spinal cord, and possibly in the brain as well, of a long-lasting group of morphine-like endorphins. Chang's research also reveals that acupuncture causes an increase in the amount of the neurotransmitter serotonin in the brain, and that this is related (in ways not yet understood) to the analgesic effects of the endorphins.[35]

These investigations into the neurophysiology of acupuncture promise to give a better understanding of the technique and its effectiveness. It has already been found that many of the traditional acupuncture points are superfluous or redundant, and some researchers are attempting to simplify the technique, and to replace the traditional meridian theory with a "segmental-innervation" theory, which is more in keeping with the new understanding of the neurochemicals.

The hypothesis that acupuncture relieves pain by stimulating the production of endorphins was tested at the Medical College of Virginia. Thirty-five volunteers were given mild electric shocks to their teeth in order to measure each individual's normal pain threshold in terms of how much electricity it took to cause pain. With the base-line established, each volunteer was treated with needles at the acupuncture point associated with tooth pain, a spot on the web between the thumb and the forefinger. After the treatment the sensitivity to pain decreased by an average of 27 percent. It took that much of an increase in electrical current to reach the threshold of pain. In order to determine whether the pain relief was due to the stimulation of endorphins, volunteers were given an injection of *naloxone,* which is known to inhibit the effects of opium and morphine, as well as the human system's natural opiates. The pain

thresholds of the volunteers injected with this substance returned to what they had been before the acupuncture treatment.[129] The indication is that some of the acupuncture
points represent the sites of "triggers" for the release of the
body's natural pain-control substances.

One of the main interests of holistic medicine is finding
means to adjust the human system's own reactions to specific
changes in the circumstances of life. The effectiveness of
acupuncture as an alternative to chemical anesthetics raises
interesting possibilities. In addition, it has been suggested that
acupuncture can modify both the stress response and the
immune response, adjusting or activating them, and prevent
the overactivity of the immune response, which can produce
such conditions as allergies and rheumatism.[6]

Modern Chinese Medicine

The World Health Organization defines health as "a state of
complete physical, mental and social well-being, not merely
the absence of disease." A utopian definition, but it is not
complete. Good health entails continual change and adjustment in one's state as conditions and demands change. Any
individual's set of health habits, and any public health system,
must be judged by its "adaptive strength," the degree to which
it assists an individual to adapt to changing conditions in the
world around him.

Chinese medicine has maintained a surprising consistency
and homogeneity of beliefs since over 2,000 years ago, when
physicians became distinct from priests and sorcerers.[51] Prevention, sanitation, and the education of physicians have always been a part of the tradition, although the central concern
has been curing disease. Substantial developments in medication and treatment occurred long before the age of modern

medicine: the use of substances containing iodine to treat goiter, ephedrine to lower blood pressure and control asthma, pomegranite rind for tapeworms. Effective treatments for the manifestations of smallpox and leprosy date back to the fourteenth century. State-supported hospitals and dispensaries date back to the ninth century, as do specialties in pediatrics, obstetrics, and gynecology.[51] Until the nineteenth century China's public health system had no rival in the West.

Also in the ninth century there developed four distinct classes of medical practitioners, which continue to the present. Medical theoreticians were at the top of the hierarchy; they were concerned most with developing and improving the overall understanding of the human system that governed both public health policies and the development and teaching of specific therapeutic techniques. Next were two classes of specialists: the part-time specialists, who were both theoreticians and practitioners, and the full-time specialists, who worked with patients as physicians, acupuncturists, masseurs, or psychological advisers. Finally there was a class of itinerant doctors, who were trained to give symptomatic and supportive therapy, and to supervise treatments ordered by the specialists.

Traditional Chinese medicine, including its diagnostic idiom, is practiced in China today primarily because it has genuine therapeutic value. The revival of acupuncture and the new official respect for it date back to the late 1950s, when "cultural nationalism" came to be supported by the political and intellectual leaders of post-revolutionary China. Formal medical education is carried out under strong central bureaucratic control. Both the physician and the paraprofessional are graduates of standardized courses in traditional medicine. Curative procedures, including the use of acupuncture and herbal remedies, continue along the same major theoretical lines established long ago, although there have been changes in specific details of the acupuncture technique in recent years.[51] At the same time, public health and preventive medicine, including inoculation and health education, operate along the lines of "cosmopolitan" modern medicine, as do surgery and ophthalmology. The two systems complement each other, and since 1958 they have officially held equal status.

In addition to physicians, with training comparable to that of a Western M.D., there are "middle doctors," who receive two or more years of practical medical training. They either assist physicians or, with further training and experience in both medical styles, establish clinics in remote areas. Finally, local "barefoot doctors," chosen by their fellow collective-farm members to receive special training, provide medical care on a part-time basis.

The barefoot doctors are trained both in Western methods of diagnosis and in the use of those traditional herbal drugs that have proven to be effective after clinical testing. As the first line of medical care, they refer cases to appropriate physicians and specialists. They examine patients when epidemiological information is being gathered, routinely deliver health care and education, practice acupuncture, dietetics, and massage, and administer drugs and medicines. Most important, they work in their own communities and treat ailments within the context of community life.[173]

Until recently, the community aspects of healing, both at the local level in specific isolated cultures and at the highly bureaucratized level exemplified by China, have been largely ignored in this country. Since the mutual recognition of China and the United States, however, the Chinese system of health care delivery has attracted particular attention.[87,98] The sharp differences between the conditions of life in China and those in the West create a situation that is ripe for the systematic study and comparison of both systems in order to determine the extent to which the multi-leveled approach to health care, education, and advice affects the overall health of the population. There is also an opportunity to sort out environmental, dietary, and behavioral factors that are related to the incidence of cancer and other diseases. It is already known that some types of cancer are more prevalent in some countries than in others. Attempts to figure out why this is the case may well provide important clues to the prevention of the disease.

CHAPTER EIGHT

Guidance from Fragmentary Information

Risk Factors

Probably the best approach to putting together a sensible, healthy way of life for yourself is to think in terms of the good things you want to include in your life rather than the bad things you want to exclude from it. We want to be free to pursue our own personal interests, to do specific things, to have specific things, to live our lives in one kind of setting rather than another. The fear of disease can become a morbid preoccupation, and it's not the sort of thing that we want to organize our lives around.

At the same time, a solid realism has to come into play about the restraints imposed on our freedom to do whatever we want to do by the facts of human nature and the facts of modern life. That means we need reliable information, so that we have a sense of where the boundaries are drawn around our freedom to choose a way of living.

Epidemiology is the systematic study of the occurrence, prevalence, and spread of disease. When infectious diseases were the main threat to human health, epidemiologists concentrated almost wholly on the question of contagion, and much of what we have come to regard as routine sanitation is the result of their tracking down the organisms that cause specific contagious diseases. The boundaries imposed on our freedom by sanitation are now so familiar that we hardly think of them.

A classic case of epidemiological detective work was carried out by a London physician, John Snow, during a cholera outbreak in 1854, in which hundreds of people died. The cause of the outbreak was a mystery, until Snow started looking for common characteristics among the victims. He found that most of them lived in one area of the city. The question then narrowed: what separated the people in this neighborhood who contracted the disease from those who didn't? Interviews revealed that the people who contracted cholera all drew their drinking water from the same public pump. The next step was to identify what differentiated that pump from others. Snow found that the pump had its source in the Thames, just downstream from a spot where raw sewage flowed into the river. Without having any clear sense of what organism caused cholera, or even the certainty that it *was* a specific organism, Snow was able to identify sewage-contaminated water as the source of the disease. It was some time afterward that the specific organism associated with cholera was identified, partly because Snow's investigation told the researchers where to look for it.

The many triumphs of public medicine over disease in the past several centuries have led us to assume that most human disorders are like cholera in that good detective work will enable us to track down the one specific agency that causes the disorder and tell us, in very certain terms, how to conquer or avoid the disease. But aside from those infectious diseases that are caused by single organisms, the causes of disease are not that simple.

There has been a shift in epidemiological studies in recent years that fits in with the overall scientific turn toward holism. The diseases that are the most common causes of death in industriaized countries are no longer the contagious diseases caused by single organisms and spread by insects or through the lack of sanitation. The big killers nowadays are heart disease, stroke, cancer, high blood pressure, and liver ailments. The causal factors of these diseases are complicated, and they cross over from one disease to another: Cigarette smoking, for example, increases the risk of both lung cancer and coronary heart disease, but both diseases are similarly related to other factors as well. "Cause" may be the wrong term for such factors; they are better understood as elements in human life associated statistically with an increase in the chance of contracting specific diseases, rather than as straightforward disease-causing agencies.

What entered into the epidemiology of the non-contagious diseases are the risk factors. Lester Breslow, dean of the School of Public Health at UCLA, divides risk factors into two groups: personal habits, such as diet, smoking, exercise, and alcohol consumption; and specific physiological changes that are precursors of disease, such as hypertension, high serum cholesterol, and certain inherited characteristics.[22] Aside from accidents or inherited tendencies or defects, the causes of serious disease are generally to be found today in the character of a person's overall adjustment to his surroundings. For the most part, your adjustment to the world is determined by what you have learned, by habits and ways of interpreting situations that have developed through a learning and conditioning process that has been going on all your life. To change it, you have to do some re-learning. Treating the results of an inadequate adjustment to the facts of modern life is a bit futile unless we pay some attention to the adjustment itself.

Imagining a perfect lifestyle is easy; the difficult part is to bridge the gap between the way things are now and the way you want them to be. Most of us cannot simply throw out a whole way of living and replace it immediately with some totally sensible alternative. We cannot ignore things like jobs, houses, and mortgages, or the other people who are involved in our daily routines.

So where do you begin? You can't just pick the disease you fear most from the list of current killers and avoid the things that cause that disease or get yourself an inoculation. Changing the habits of your life so as to minimize the risk of disease means first identifying those personal characteristics associated with disease that you can do something about. But reliable, straightforward information on such matters is difficult to find.

What You Read in the Papers

Common sense tells you that the foods you eat, the amount of rest and exercise you get, the kinds of stress you experience at work and at home, and many other factors have something to do with how well you feel. The problem is, how can we make sound judgments about these things? Life just isn't what it used to be. Better in some ways, worse in others, but *different* in many respects from one decade to another. The common wisdom of one generation is the old-fogeyism of the next. Even the medical experts don't agree among themselves, so it's hard to know whom to listen to.

Because we are all concerned about cancer, every little

snippet of information about cancer research becomes news. We read in the morning paper that the Japanese, who eat a lot of smoked fish, have a high incidence of stomach cancer. We give up smoked fish. A few weeks later, we hear an interview with a researcher who suspects that smoked fish is harmless if we get plenty of vitamin C. So we drink grapefruit juice with smoked fish. Then another bit of information and another reason to modify our habits comes along. It can become silly, and we begin to wish that medical research would get together and give us some concrete, conclusive, definitive recommendations.

Nutrition in particular is controversial. Most doctors recommend a balanced diet, perhaps supplemented with a good multivitamin. But researchers in nutrition say that doctors were never trained in nutrition; it has been almost wholly neglected in medical schools.[182] The researcher has his own ideas about the amount of vitamins and minerals we require, and it conflicts with the doctor's advice. The doctor, in turn, says that the nutritionist's advice is still just a hypothesis; it hasn't been demonstrated.

Part of the problem is that we have *too much* raw information thrown at us in press reports of specific studies. What we need, but don't get, is the overall picture, and we need to know about the methods of medical research, the assumptions that researchers make, and the biases that they have.

The classic way to establish a scientific hypothesis is by controlled experiment. You set up a laboratory situation in such a way as to isolate just the items you want to study, and artificially hold all other items at some constant state. You might, for example, take two groups of laboratory animals which are as alike genetically as you can manage, cage them in the same way, keep the temperature, humidity, and the periods of light and darkness the same for both groups, and feed them the same diet except for one substance, X. Then after a period of time you note the differences between the two groups, and you can state with confidence that the differences are due to that one X factor.

Well, you just can't do that kind of controlled experiment with human beings. No two of us are alike genetically, except for identical twins. Even in the same household, no two of us have exactly the same daily habits, the same emotional relationships with other people, the same diets, the same pressures and responsibilities. We can't separate out X factors one at a time; there are just too many variables that differentiate one person from another.

One way to iron out the individual differences among people and try to identify the effect of specific factors on health is to go in the opposite direction from controlled experiment and conduct statistical studies on entire populations in their natural settings. This seldom yields straightforward information about which factors cause what conditions, but it does yield clues to the role of specific factors in human health.

Some years ago, a French nutritionist studied populations who lived in areas where the soil was depleted in the mineral zinc. Presumably the vegetables and the food for livestock grown and eaten in the region would be lower than normal in zinc, and so the amount of zinc in the overall diet would be lower for these people than for those who lived in areas where the soil was rich in zinc. How would the two groups differ in quality of health? The most easily available figures are those that show the causes of death. So the question is this: Is there a significant difference in the causes of death between the people who live in zinc-depleted areas and those who live in zinc-rich areas?

What emerged from the study is that populations who live in zinc-poor areas have statistically higher suicide rates than populations who live in areas where the level of zinc in the soil (and the local diet) is higher.[37]

Suicide? How could suicide be connected with the level of zinc in the diet? The correlation stood up in a number of geographically scattered areas where the geological surveys showed zinc-depleted soils. But no researcher is going to claim that a deficiency in zinc causes suicide. That strains the limits of plausibility. The connection must be indirect, and it involves making assumptions about the *possibility* of connections existing between diet and physiological states, between physiological and emotional states, and finally, between emotional states—depression or instability—and the likelihood of suicide. Nevertheless, the statistical correlation is an interesting clue to be followed up.

At the University of Michigan, samples of students' hair were examined and analyzed for the presence of trace minerals, including zinc. (Analyzing hair samples is an easy and painless way to estimate the levels of specific minerals in the system.) The students who showed the highest levels of zinc and copper were also those who had the highest academic grades. Another clue? Surely, the connection must have to do with intellectual functioning. Combining the suicide clue and the academic clue, however, might indicate a connection between the presence of zinc in the body and the function of the neuroregulators in the brain, perhaps those affecting mood, stability, or the ability to concentrate.

More evidence: Children with zinc-deficient diets have slow growth rates, poor appetites, and senses of taste and smell that are less acute than normal. Following up this clue, some researchers added zinc supplements to the diets of adult patients whose senses of taste and smell were impaired. Sensory impairment of that sort has always been difficult to treat, and most often it has been approached as a psychiatric problem. But 103 patients who were given the zinc supplement recovered their senses of taste and smell.[37]

Can we explain the connection on a physiological level?

Here is where the biochemists come in, but the information is spotty. The exact role of zinc in the system is not known; the medical literature is filled with well-hedged statements about what the role of zinc *might* be in certain functions, or what its *probable* role is in others. Clearly zinc is essential to the functioning of cells and in the structure of cell membranes, and it seems to be important in the synthesis of the all-important nucleic acids DNA and RNA. It also figures in many of the processes involved in the action of white blood cells in the immune response.[34] It is important also in the synthesis of neuroregulators, and it is essential for the proper functioning of the male sexual system. But few of those functions of zinc in the human system are understood in detail. Statistical studies indicate the importance of zinc in the diet and at the same time provide a guide for the biochemists who are trying to establish just how the element functions in our cells.

Studies of the incidence of disease in domestic animals can provide information as well. Leukemia in cattle is prevalent in areas where the soil is depleted in magnesium. In Poland, cattle in the intensively farmed northern section of the country have a much higher incidence of leukemia than cattle in the southern sections, where farming has been carried out by less modern and less intensive methods. Leukemia in human beings has increased sharply in some parts of the country since 1960, but *not* in areas where the soil and the drinking water have a high content of magnesium.[186] That is strong evidence that deficiencies in magnesium increase susceptibility to the disease. Follow-up studies with laboratory animals bear out the findings. One's first impulse might be to add huge amounts of magnesium to the daily diet. Perhaps magnesium is the magic substance that will prevent leukemia and other cancers. But it isn't that simple. There are no such magic substances. And worse yet, animal studies show that once a colony of cancerous cells is well established, magnesium and potassium encourage its growth.[120]

Specific nutrients have been found to be effective in the treatment of disorders in large "mega" doses. But interrelations among the nutrients make it imprudent to react too quickly to those isolated reports. Magnesium, for example, can be utilized in the system only if it is in a certain balance with calcium. The daily intake of calcium should be about two and a half times that of magnesium. But many people don't receive the minerals in these proportions. A study of the meals served in college dining halls showed that the amount of calcium supplied was five times as much as the amount of magnesium—twice the proportion required to keep the two in balance. Moreover, the supply of magnesium was about 250 milligrams per day, whereas the Recommended Daily Allowance, a conservative estimate of the requirement of the nutrient in the diet, calls for 350 milligrams per day.

We need a number of different minerals in small but balanced amounts in order to function properly. The most familiar is iron, which figures in the production of red blood cells. We receive guidance from nutritionists about avoiding deficiencies by taking dietary supplements or by choosing foods carefully. For iron, eat your spinach and liver; for zinc, include seafood in your diet or increase the amount of seeds and nuts; for magnesium, eat whole grains, spinach, corn, nuts, and legumes, such as peas or lima beans. However, these bits of good advice are unsatisfying in their lack of directness about cause-and-effect relationships between diet and health.

Those neat cause-and-effect relationships don't exist for some diseases. No one magic mineral will keep you from getting cancer or heart disease or rheumatoid arthritis. The conditions that lead to them are too complex to yield to that kind of approach. So we come back to risk factors. How can you be *sure* that you won't develop cancer or heart disease? You can't. All you can do is try to *minimize* the risk. And we're back to the problem of getting reliable guidance and information about how to lead a healthy life.

Much of the information connecting diet and the incidence of disease has come from the intense involvement of the medical profession with attempts to pin down the conditions that lead to cancer. Tracking down dietary clues to these conditions involves gathering two sets of statistics: the per-capita consumption of specific kinds of food in given countries or regions, and the incidence of specific diseases. Information isn't available for a good part of the world, although the National Cancer Institute and other research organizations and governments are pressing hard to get such information on a county-by-county basis in the United States, and in as much detail as possible from other countries as well. The more detailed statistical information we have on a variety of human populations, the more clues we are likely to find concerning what makes the difference in the incidence of disease from one population to another. But they are *just* clues, and they are about events on the level of whole populations, not about events that involve individuals.

Here is a good case of statistical detective work. The United States, Scotland, New Zealand, Canada, and Denmark, the countries with the highest per-capita consumption of beef, which is very rich in fat, also have the highest per-capita incidence of intestinal cancer. Is there a connection? One statistical correlation doesn't establish it. The next step is to look at countries where the per-capita consumption of animal fats is particularly low, such as Japan. The incidence of intestinal cancer in Japan is less than 27 percent of that in the United States. But that still doesn't make the point; surely the typical lifestyle in Japan differs from ours in many other ways. Moreover, the populations with high incidence of intestinal cancer are predominantly Caucasian. So more clues must be found. Japanese-Americans who have adopted the American eating habits, high in beef and butter, have about the same incidence of the disease as other Americans. So it isn't just a matter of race. That makes the dietary connection more likely, but it still doesn't clinch the case. (In fact, nothing would clinch the case absolutely except the kinds of controlled experiment that we just can't do on live human beings.)

Is there a population of Caucasian Americans who don't eat much beef? Seventh-Day Adventists are mostly Caucasian, and a good many are vegetarians. And they do have a lower rate of intestinal cancer than the overall American population. This is a good *prima facie* case for a connection between the consumption of animal fats and the incidence of the disease on a *population level*. But you and I are not populations; we are individuals. Not every beef-eating American gets intestinal cancer, and not every fish-eating Japanese avoids it.

Two questions must be answered, then. First, *how* is the consumption of animal fats connected with the development of intestinal cancer? One likely hypothesis is that while fats are being digested they stimulate both digestive substances and bacteria that interact to form carcinogens. The second question goes back to population studies. What is it that differentiates those beef-eaters who get the disease from those who don't? One country for which figures are available and in which the consumption of animal fats is high and the incidence of intestinal cancer is low is Finland. What sets the Finns apart? Their diet differs from those in the high-incidence countries primarily in the large amount of fiber they consume, such as whole-grain breads and bran.

How does this guide us in choosing our foods? We know that cancer is a complex disease, that dozens of factors are involved in the development of uncontrolled colonies of abnormal cells in the body, ranging from emotional factors and inherited characteristics to overall nourishment. Obviously, animal fats alone don't cause cancer, but they can play a part.

So such studies do offer some guidance: consume less fat and more fiber, and diversify your diet so that it doesn't become overbalanced with one particular kind of food.

Laboratory Animals and You

There is always some argument about the use of laboratory animals in detecting the causes of human diseases, and the arguments have become particularly intense in recent years because from time to time public health agencies have banned or restricted the use of particular substances which have produced cancer in animals.

How seriously should we take animal studies? If a certain percentage of laboratory animals develops bladder cancer when fed absurdly huge amounts of artificial sweeteners, does it have anything to do with us? In the absence of any better indicators, *yes.* It comes down to a question of where we can find the best available evidence as to which substances are likely to increase the number of mutations in human cells. The aim of the enormous doses is not to reproduce a human situation but to establish whether or not there is any relationship at all between the concentration of the substance and the development of malignant tumors. Of course, as the counter-argument goes, *any* substance will kill laboratory animals at some level of concentration. The question is, which ones will kill them of *cancer,* and at what concentrations? The public health argument, which some people question, is that if increasingly large doses of a chemical will cause an increase in tumors in laboratory animals in a short period, than there is good reason to believe that smaller doses over a longer period will cause tumors as well. In most cases where such connections have been tested, the argument has been borne out.

As much as laboratory animals differ from human beings, the attempt is made in such studies to use animals whose systems or organs most closely resemble those of human beings. Donald Kennedy, a biologist who served as Commissioner of the Food and Drug Administration from 1977 to 1979 argues:

> We learn that beneath the remarkable array of living forms is an equally remarkable similarity of process in the extraction of energy from the environment, in the chemistry of inheritance, in the control of growth. Evolution, so radical in generating new forms of life, was extremely conservative with these basic processes. There is every reason to believe that cancer is an example of basic processes gone awry. The similarities between cancer in animals and in human beings . . . are powerful arguments for the appropriateness of using animals as models for people.[86]

Eighteen substances known to be carcinogens in human beings were tested on laboratory animals; sixteen were carcinogenic in the animals. But of the substances that prove to be carcinogenicer first in animal studies, only a few have been subsequently observed directly in human populations. Researchers can study asbestos workers, the neighbors of the Three-Mile Island accident, and the inhabitants of the chemically polluted Love Canal region, but unless there is a population of human beings already exposed to a substance by virtue of occupation, accident, or other fact of human life, researchers cannot create one. In the absence of direct human tests, and in the absence of epidemiological evidence based on occupational or other exposure, animal studies constitute the best available evidence concerning the carcinogenic properties of specific substances. Other biochemical tests under development promise to give a measure of a substance's mutagenic properties in specific kinds of tissue. These involve the study of tissue cultures rather than live animals or people, but they are still under development. We'll hear more about them when the critical consensus in the medical community is strong enough that they are generally regarded as reliable.

Another way to determine whether or not the more than 50,000 man-made chemicals currently in commercial and industrial use are likely to be carcinogenic is to measure the ability of a substance to cause mutations in bacteria by means of the Ames Test and other related procedures.[3] Such tests are considerably faster and less expensive than tests on laboratory animals. And the kind of damage that chemicals can do to the genetic material of human cells is similar to the kind of damage they can do to bacteria. When the bacterial tests were evaluated by trying them with substances already known to be carcinogenic or non-carcinogenic, they were able to distinguish the two groups of substances with 90-percent accuracy. In addition, the bacterial tests identified some substances as potential carcinogens that were later shown to be carcinogenic in animal tests.[44]

Meanwhile, the argument goes on about the reliability of information based on animal testing and epidemiological evidence. Remember that science never deals with matters that are subject to ultimate proof, only with hypotheses that either do or do not stand up to criticism and experimental testing. I think it is fair to say that the consensus of the scientific community is that animal tests provide the best available evidence of cancer hazards at present, with the faster but slightly less reliable bacterial tests running a close second.

Even if we had the complete list of known carcinogens, we would obviously not be able to avoid every one. We can only minimize their presence. However, those carcinogens that can overwhelm even the strongest immune system might be avoided altogether. Asbestos and vinyl chloride are two such substances. And it is sensible to insist that asbestos paneling be removed from office buildings and schools, and that another kind of insulation be found for hair dryers and toasters.

In general, the best guidance is to avoid so far as possible those substances that are judged to be hazardous on the basis of the best available evidence, recognizing that some mistakes will be made.

The saccharine controversy is a case in point. In a study done in Canada in 1974, one hundred rats were saturated with saccharine. Their diet consisted of 5 percent pure saccharine, beginning not with their birth, but with their mother's diets from *conception* on through their birth, life, and death. Another group of one hundred animals received no saccharine at all. Fourteen of the saccharine-saturated rats had developed bladder tumors by the time they died; only two of the control group had. Never mind how many diet colas you'd have to drink over the course of a lifetime to match that consumption of saccharine; that's not the point. The point is that at *some* concentration, the saccharine was implicated in the development of cancer in 12 percent of an animal population.

There are two additional steps required in this line of reasoning, to take us from the results of the animal tests to the conclusion that we should avoid saccharine. First, it needs to be argued that a lesser amount of saccharine would still have produced a significant but proportionally smaller number of bladder cancers in the animals (and this is probably so); second, it must be argued that what holds for the animals holds for human beings as well. It is the second step that has stirred up controversy, although the argument has held up in other cases. In subsequent studies, researchers turned to the medical records of diabetics, who consume considerably more saccharine than most people do. The incidence of bladder cancer was not significantly greater than that of the public at large. Further studies with rhesus monkeys (which are more closely related to human beings than the rats used in the original study) showed no incidence of bladder cancer over a six-year period. But more recent human studies confirm that there is a weak connection after all, and the Food and Drug Administration has acted to limit the use of the substance. The consensus of public health authorities is that saccharine is indeed implicated in the incidence of bladder cancer. That's the difficulty with best available evidence: it changes; it is rarely final. Over a period of time, as the evidence changes, reasonable decisions must be revised.

The use of saccharine is still a matter of some debate, despite the more recent studies and the FDA's move to regulate the substance. For many people, the alternative to saccharine is sugar, which in some cases may provide an even higher risk of disease. The *most* prudent thing to do, whether or not the dispute continues, is to avoid the substance altogether. If it is used at all, it should be used sparingly.

Minimizing Risk Factors

What we know about specific *combinations* of risk factors and the risk of disease is even more sketchy than what we know about specific individual factors. The few available studies of combined hazards indicate that the results of two apparently unrelated habits of life occurring in combination can materially increase disease risks. For example, moderate smokers who are heavy drinkers are twenty-five times more likely to develop cancer of the esophagus than moderate smokers who never drink.[86]

We clearly need information about combined risk factors, but studies with human populations are devilishly difficult to devise and arrange. A two-year study in heart-disease prevention carried out by Stanford University involved three northern California towns, each with a population between 12,000 and 15,000. The towns were surveyed to find out how much people knew about health risks and to get a set of base-line figures about the local habits of behavior related to diet, smoking, exercise, and weight. A sample of each population was given a medical examination and an interview to determine health habits. The first town was kept as a control; nothing more was done until two years later. The second town was subjected to a blitzkrieg of multimedia information, including hour-long radio and television programs about diet, smoking, and exercise, radio spot advertisements, newspaper advertisements and feature stories, billboards, posters, and direct mailings of information about health care. The third community got the multimedia blitz *plus* personal instruction for a random sample of that 25 percent of the population who were considered to have the highest risk of heart disease on the basis of measurable physiological variables like blood pressure and serum cholesterol.

At the end of each of the two years, the communities were surveyed again, and the changes in both physiological states related to heart disease and the overall reported habits of the population were noted. In the two communities that had received the information campaign, the risk of coronary heart disease had declined 15 percent to 20 percent over the two-year period. In the control community, which did not receive the informational blitz, the risk of coronary heart disease had actually *increased* by more than 5 percent. In the groups that received personal instruction, the decline of risk was about 30 percent. Specific measures, such as the consumption of saturated fat and cholesterol, and measurements of serum cholesterol in the blood, showed an even more notable change: 20 to 40 percent over the two-year period in the communities where the campaign was conducted. Smoking decreased by 7 percent to 24 percent in those communities, compared to only 2.5 percent in the control community; and among those who received intensive instruction, the drop in smoking was 42 percent.[53, 102]

The study indicates that the measurable risk of heart disease, cancer, and other diseases related to the habits of modern life can be changed for the better if people are informed of the risks and how to deal with them.

A study carried out in high-risk communities in northern Finland produced similar results. By providing public health information, organizing community health services to deal with people's habits and behavior as well as their clinical symptoms, restricting cigarette smoking in public places, and providing detailed information about self-care to people who already had clinical symptoms, the annual incidence of strokes was cut in half. Forty percent of the population showed a decrease of at least 10 points in systolic blood pressure. And the habits associated with risk—the consumption of fats, cigarette smoking, and so on—were adjusted to an extent much like that of the Stanford study.[22] Dealing with these risk factors—diet, cigarette smoking, alcohol consumption, rest, exercise, and weight control—is as much a matter of personal and public hygiene as sanitation, sewage disposal, and food handling are. If the direct causal links between these risk factors and specific diseases aren't clear, there is at least as good a case for their relevance to the incidence of disease as there was for the relevance of sewage-contaminated drinking water to the 1854 cholera outbreak.

The risk factors involved in the Stanford study are all connected with the non-infectious "diseases of civilization." The major additional factor in these diseases is stress. A study carried out by William Meecham of the UCLA School of Engineering and Applied Science found that the 80,000 people who live within a three-mile radius of Los Angeles International Airport have a 19 percent higher overall death rate than people who live six miles away. Most of the difference was a result of stress-related diseases. The group close to the airport had 40 percent more fatal strokes and 140 percent more deaths from cirrhosis of the liver than the control group. There is no reason to suppose that these frightening differences in people's health are directly caused by the noise of jets passing over the area, but as Meecham notes, the diseases involved seem to be hurried along by the resulting tension.[161]

In less dramatic, less measurable ways, each of us is affected by the noises, tensions, and demands of modern life, and we need to deal with those risk factors as part of an overall program of personal care and hygiene. Moving further away from the airport is one way to do it, but those noises, tensions, and demands cannot be eliminated altogether. Modern society puts us in constant contact with them. So if we can't avoid them, we have to learn to deal with them and develop ways to lessen their effects.

CHAPTER NINE

Dealing with Stress

Biofeedback: The Voluntary and the Involuntary

Every day we perform unconsciously coordinated actions like driving a car, playing a piano, or typing a letter. In the ordinary course of events, we don't pay attention to how we do these things once we have learned them, unless we decide that there is something wrong with the *way* we do them. Then we work on the technique itself, paying attention to what we do and taking conscious control over the activity so that we can correct whatever it is that's wrong. Such ordinarily unconscious activities can be "made conscious" again, and the habits of activity deliberately changed.

We can do the same thing in many cases involving unconscious biological activity. Breathing, for instance, is unconscious unless we experience some discomfort or irregularity, or unless we are, say, trying to keep our presence in a room secret from someone else. But when the occasion demands it, we can speed up or slow down our breathing, take in great gulps of air and expel them with enormous force or, sitting quietly, deliberately make our breathing shallow and silent. You can control your breathing because there are clear-cut sensations associated with it. You can *feel* yourself breathe, and you can change the rate and depth of your breath because you can tell from the feeling just how it is going. But you can't feel your blood pressure, or the rate at which you digest food. You aren't ordinarily aware of the rate of your heartbeat unless it is outside comfortable ranges. The signals aren't there.

Until about 1970, Western physiologists thought they could make sharp distinctions between those activities that we could control consciously and those that we couldn't. The autonomic nervous system maintains the economy of the system; it regulates heartbeat, breathing rate, the opening and narrowing of specific blood vessels, blood pressure, the production of hormones, the peristaltic movements of the intestines in digesting food, the levels of moisture on the skin, the levels of acid in the stomach, and so on. Few clear-cut signals indicate changes in functions like these unless something is really wrong. *Autonomic* came to be understood as *automatic,* not subject to conscious control.

Then in the 1960s came the technology of *biofeedback.* The physiologists were wrong, we were told; we *can* control many of our inner states; the conception of automatic biological processes that we all learned in school was dead wrong. The reaction of much of the medical community was predictable and essentially conservative. Another useless gimmick, they told us; the only reliable way to control blood pressure is with medication; it is impossible just to decide how the autonomic nervous system is going to function. Both extremes have been pretty well discredited by experiments with biofeedback since the inflated claims first appeared. We can indeed bring far more of our physiological functions under conscious control than was previously thought possible. We can't take over *every* physiological function, and if we could we wouldn't have time to think about anything else. As Lewis Thomas suggests, the business of the liver is best left to the liver.[170] Like driving and typing, the details of these activities are better suppressed so that you can save your conscious attention for the things you need to do each day. But again, like driving and typing, there might be good reason in specific cases to pay attention to activities that are ordinarily unconscious so that you can change the habits surrounding them and *then* let the whole thing slip back to unconscious regulation with some bad habits corrected.

The premise of biofeedback is quite simple: if we can get a clear and unambiguous signal to indicate when a given function is in a desired state, then we may be able to learn to control that function and to change the unconscious habits connected with it. This involves some form of sensing device that will produce a signal—an audible tone or a flashing light—when the function is within the desired limits. Effectively, you learn to maintain the signal which is linked to the sensing equipment.

Suppose you want to maintain your systolic blood pressure below, say, 130. A device to measure the blood pressure, hooked up to a signal source, will indicate when the blood pressure falls below 130. The aim is to maintain the tone, and with practice, you can.

How do you do it? That's another question. But then how do you control your breathing? Unless you are a professional singer, you are probably not aware of how you control your breathing, or which muscles you use. You just *do* it, and you have clear sensations to indicate how it's going. In the case of blood pressure and other functions, the gadgetry gives you the appropriate signals. Even laboratory animals can be trained to control such functions in surprisingly precise ways by means of biofeedback equipment and conditioning techniques. If a rat can be taught to increase the blood circulation to its left ear while keeping the circulation in the right ear constant, then you and I can certainly learn to do similar, but more useful things.[45]

Participants in a study designed to teach the control of heartbeat were surprised to learn just how variable the heart rate is. The slightest muscle movement or change in breathing affects the rate. But there are far less direct ways to affect it. Think about walking along a quiet path in the woods and the heartbeat slows down; think about doing your income tax or having a nasty argument with a friend and it speeds up again. Still more subtle connections can be made: imagine warmth or heaviness in the area of the heart, and it will slow down; imagine lightness or constriction and it accelerates.[69]

In the laboratory and in clinical situations, most people can learn to control their blood pressure, heart rate, the level of moisture on the skin, the blood circulation to specific parts of the body (warming one hand but not the other, for example), brain activity, muscle tension, even the level of stomach acidity and the white blood cell count.[23, 69] Even more encouraging, some patients with paralysis resulting from stroke or other neural damage have been able to re-learn specific muscle functions. If the natural sensations connected with bodily movement are cut off, they can be replaced in some cases with biofeedback equipment that shows how muscles are functioning and teaches patients how to regain control of lost functions.[23] Patients with epilepsy have been able to normalize their brain waves and reduce the incidence of seizures.[163, 164] And patients with migraine or Raynaud's disease have been taught how to alter the patterns of blood circulation and thus alleviate attacks.

The biofeedback experiments demonstrate that control over our own states is possible. The demonstration has been carried out in public and testable ways, and the medical professions have had to think again about the nature of the autonomic nervous system. Hans Selye, who brought the biologic aspects of stress into the medical literature twenty years ago, sees biofeedback as a means for controlling stress by bringing into awareness the indices of stress that are reflected in the measured and signaled states: heart rate, blood pressure, muscular tension, brain-wave patterns, and so on.[147]

The difficulty comes when we try to take these effects out of the laboratory. People just can't carry thousands of dollars worth of electronic equipment with them all the time to make sure that their blood pressure is where they want it to be. Even if they could, listening for that signal all day long would be such a distraction that nothing else would get done.

Dr. Lester Fehmi, a psychologist who directs a biofeedback clinic in Princeton, New Jersey, believes that biofeedback is one of the most important medical developments in history. I asked him how he deals with the problem of taking the positive results of biofeedback out of the laboratory and into his patients' daily lives. His answer was: "I cheat."

A clinical situation, where biofeedback is used to help someone with a problem, is different from a research situation, where the aim is to determine whether or not control over bodily states can actually be accomplished. Coaching, suggestion, or instruction would contaminate a research design; they really would constitute cheating. But they are often the difference between a sterile exercise and genuine help for a patient in a clinical situation, as they are for any patient in any clinical situation.

Fehmi's "cheating" consists of introducing his patients to a combination of techniques designed to help them maintain the physiological states they have learned to achieve with the monitoring equipment. Fehmi borrows freely from hypnosis, meditation and Zen in order to help his patients take out of the biofeedback laboratory what they have learned there. Part of the cheating involves a peculiar use of words.

When Westerners hear words and sentences, especially in a medical context, we expect them to make sense. When they don't make sense, we suspect that something is fishy. A lot of nonsense has been foisted on the gullible for generations, and much of it has been presented as part of the "Mysteries of the East." There has been enough fakery in the past that we are justifiably suspicious.

But there is an alternative between sense and nonsense. Sometimes we do things that *might* be meant to convey information, but clearly aren't. A pianist who does finger exercises while riding on a bus might be confused with someone using sign language or making obscene gestures. If you were to ask what his finger exercises *mean,* it would be like asking for the meaning of a push-up. Even the people who talk about "body language" wouldn't ask about push-ups, because push-ups don't mean anything. They are exercises, and the reason for doing them has nothing to do with conveying a meaning.

Sometimes we do the same thing with words. If a child comes home from school and says that he has been told by the speech teacher to say "She sells sea shells by the sea shore" as fast as he can without messing it up, and to do this at least twenty times every day, you aren't going to ask about what sort of seashells she sells, or how many shekels she sells them for, or whether the sheriff suspects that she sells surreptitiously synthesized specious seashells to susceptible citizens. The sentence is clearly an exercise. Meaning has nothing to do with it. Language does not function cognitively in it.

So it is with the koan. Koans aren't *supposed* to mean anything. They don't in any literal way make sense. They are a peculiar kind of exercise, typically in the form of questions, not designed to improve muscle control, but to elicit a specific response nonetheless. Probably the most familiar koan from the Zen tradition is the question "What is the sound of one hand clapping?" Of course, the question doesn't make sense. Beyond that, this particular koan has become a tired cliché.

But can you imagine the distance between your eyes? Is it possible for you to imagine the volume of your fingers? Take this seriously now. Is it possible for you to imagine the space inside your throat? Can you imagine the distance between the space inside your throat and the top of your head?

Lester Fehmi asks his patients these questions and others like them in the course of what he calls Open Focus training.

The questions aren't meant to be answered. What matters is the effect the question has on the patient. The questions are designed to direct the subject's imagination to what Fehmi calls an "objectless image," such as distance, space, and volume. The patient is never directed to think about anything, but only asked if he *can* think about it. Attention is diffused over a region of space, rather than focused sharply on an object, hence the term *open focus*.

If this seems like a simple-minded or pointless exercise, it is partly because we expect to give concrete answers to questions. The answer, in this case, isn't articulated; but the response *can* be measured as a change in physiological states. Once his subjects learn how to listen to the questions, Fehmi asks questions and monitors responses for a full hour. Later, the time per session is cut to a half hour or less, while the patient listens to recorded questions. The result? A measurable increase in the amplitude of alpha activity in individual lobes of the brain, and in the synchrony of this activity among the lobes. This is an accepted clinical sign of a state of unstressed relaxation. Moreover, the hands become warm, indicating an unobstructed blood flow; the muscle tension decreases; and perhaps more significant, if the blood pressure has been elevated, it decreases toward normal levels.[54]

Most important of all, exercises like these can be done at home with only a tape-cassette player; and after a short time most subjects can practice with no equipment at all. As Fehmi explains:

> After repeated practice, patients can often enter a
> state of Open Focus without actually going through the
> exercises, but simply by reminding themselves of that state
> through the use of a cue word or phrase, such as "Open
> Focus." This phenomenon appears analogous to the
> situation in which even the thought of a stimulus or event
> evokes the associated effect and state of mind.[54]

The important thing about Fehmi's Open Focus and similar techniques is that they work, and they needn't be applied only in a laboratory setting. In some clinical situations, patients can learn to control by themselves what previously had to be controlled with medication or extended therapy. Thus a new standard of patient's responsibility is developing, with medical *guidance* rather than direct medical *treatment*.

The Relaxation Response

Beginning in the late 1950s, physiologists from the United States and India, using portable equipment, measured the electrical activity of the brain, heart, and skeletal muscles of Indian yogis during their traditional meditations.[5, 179] Specific claims for spectacular effects were tested: the ability to make the heart appear to stop, to induce sweating at will, to control bleeding, and to slow down the metabolism of the whole system to such an extent that the yogi could simulate death. The more interesting, if less dramatic, achievements from a medical point of view were the effects on blood pressure, which was lowered during meditation; electrical activity in the brain, which displayed a strong "alpha" pattern associated with deep relaxation while awake; increased electrical resistance in the skin, a sign of diminished anxiety; and a general decrease in muscle tension. Later studies of Zen meditators in Japan showed similar results.[83] It became clear that the psychological techniques developed in the Eastern meditative traditions could produce the kind of control over physiological states that was being sought in the West by means of biofeedback equipment.[121]

Because most of the techniques used to overcome the effects of stress are borrowed from Oriental traditions of medicine and self-discipline, they strike many Westerners as mystical and alien. When a Westerner hears the word "mysticism," he thinks of unscientific lore, the occult—literally the "hidden" things of the world. To Orientals, mysticism means *experience,* but in a way that seems incomprehensible to us because it often means the kind of experience that is not easily described and therefore not easily dealt with scientifically. The impediment to a clearer understanding of such experience has been the artificial and misleading distinction between the occult—hidden—mind, and the mechanical—public—body that has been driven so deeply into the very structure of the language we in the West use to describe ourselves.

Until recently, the two traditions of science, Eastern and Western, existed separately because of geographical distance, and they were thought to be incommensurable. The Eastern tradition studied human beings first, and did that by means of a psychology of experience. The Western tradition tried to set the objects of study apart from human experience, to study them at a distance by means of a physics and a physically oriented study of living processes. But the geographical barriers have been overcome, and so have the conceptual barriers. There is now the possibility of a truly global human science that can combine the best insights of both traditions.[157]

The study of perception, emotion, and learning from the point of view of individual experience rather than that of overt behavior poses difficult problems in experimental design and theoretical articulation. What has come to be called the "psychology of consciousness"[118] combines the experience-oriented theory and technique of the Eastern psychologies and the behavior-oriented psychologies of the West. The altered states of consciousness associated with meditation provide a way of getting at the synthesis. Like the attempt to study the framework of beliefs, expectations, and individual orientation that enter into perception from the phenomenological point of view, the attempt to study different modes of consciousness and awareness is just beginning in a serious way. The direction is pointed to a broader conception of what counts as "normal" human experience, but the theoretical and experimental work is still in its early stages.

Meanwhile, the medical and physiological aspects of the convergence of traditions is progressing, as Western scientists are attempting to understand not only meditative techniques, but the theoretical traditions in which they developed. Western research in this area has come to be known as the study of the *relaxation response*,[17] understood now as a natural set of activities in the brain, nervous system, and other organs that is as firmly ingrained in our biological makeup as is the stress response, studied by Hans Selye.

In 1968 Herbert Benson and his colleagues at Harvard University Medical School were studying monkeys to determine connections between specific patterns of behavior and blood pressure. As news of the work got around, the researchers were approached by a group of students who were practicing Transcendental Meditation, a simplified yoga technique that had been popularized by the Beatles and their teacher, the Maharishi Mahesh Yogi. The students wanted Benson and his group to use *them* in the studies of behavior and blood pressure, so that the claimed benefits of TM could be put to a test by researchers who had no stake in the outcome.

Benson agreed, and he soon discovered that studies were also being carried out at UCLA by R. Keith Wallace as part of his research on a doctoral dissertation under the guidance of Dr. Archie K. Wilson. (Wallace and Benson eventually worked together and published some of their results jointly.[177])

At the outset the researchers needed to establish what meditation *isn't*. If meditation were just a matter of being half-asleep or hypnotized, or in some other well-understood state, then their research would have to take a different direction than if it were something new and relatively unstudied. But they determined that it was neither sleep nor hypnosis, and further, that it did not resemble hibernation. The meditative state is measurably distinct: Electrical activity in the brain, measurable metabolic functions such as oxygen consumption, and the levels of lactate and other substances in the blood all show somewhat different patterns in sleep than they do in meditation; and the states in hypnosis vary widely according to what is suggested.

What Benson and his colleagues discovered about the physiology of meditation has been well publicized by TM proponents. During meditation the rate of metabolism decreases measurably. Breathing slows down, less oxygen is taken in, less carbon dioxide is exhaled without any detectable change in the amount of oxygen in the blood. The system isn't starving for oxygen, it is *using* less, and this indicates a general relaxation of the pace of bodily processes. At the same time, the heart rate slows, muscle tension decreases, and if the blood pressure has been elevated, it decreases. And there are more subtle indicators of a general state of relaxation and freedom from stress: Alpha activity increases, indicating a resting state; and the level of lactate in the blood, which is high during states of anxiety and emotional arousal, drops significantly during the first ten minutes of meditation. Benson also found a carryover effect: People who meditate regularly show a gradually increasing state of overall relaxation and freedom from tension. Now that's a highly desirable package of effects to be able to achieve all by yourself. The set of responses is as well organized as the fight-or-flight response, and it provides a way to break the pattern of generally harmful effects that stress generates.

The combination of effects observed in meditation is a well-established natural biological response for protecting an individual against the harmful effects of the fight-or-flight response. The same combination is grouped together in other animals as well. Benson cites the work of Walter R. Hess, a Nobel Laureate in physiology. Working with cats, Hess found the trigger for the fight-or-flight response by stimulating one area of the hypothalamus. By stimulating another area, an opposite sort of response was initiated, one that acted as a protective measure against overstress and promoted the restoration of the system from the demands of stress. This second response, which Hess called *trophotropic,* involves physiologic changes similar to those Benson and his colleagues observed in the meditators. It is the kind of state a cat goes into when it sits quietly, purring.

The true value of this response, according to Lester Fehmi, is that it allows the homeostatic tendency of the human system to heal and balance the body chemistry. The relaxation response decreases the activity of the autonomic nervous system and restores order. One probable explanation for the generation of this natural response through meditation is that meditation diminishes the stimuli to the thalamus by means of an inward focus and a general passive, relaxed state of *letting* things happen, rather than forcing them to happen. The thalamus returns to its natural rhythm, without stimulation, and that in turn seems to affect the hypothalamus region, which is where Dr. Hess found the trigger for the corresponding response in the cats.

The connection between the fight-or-flight response and the relaxation response is striking. All the measurable bodily states that increase in the fight-or-flight response—oxygen consumption, heart rate, respiratory rate, blood pressure, and so on—decrease with the relaxation response. But what triggers this response? Is it peculiar to one form or another of meditation, or can it be initiated without using any specific technique? And if it is a natural biological response, why haven't we been aware of it before?

Benson argues that almost every human culture *has* been

aware of the relaxation response, typically in the form of a religious exercise. He cites passages from the Upanishads, part of the Vedic literature dating from the sixth century B.C., which formed the background for the Maharashi Mahesh Yogi's system of meditation. The basic elements of meditation are also described in Brahmanism, Hinduism, Buddhism, and Taoism, and by Confucius, the Japanese Zen masters, by such Christian mystics as St. Augustine and St. Térèse, and such Jewish mystics as Rabbi Abulafia. Even the American "nature mystics" Henry David Thoreau and Ralph Waldo Emerson used the same basic technique in relaxation and contemplation. As Benson says, it seems that everybody knows it but us, and in our stress-generating Western society, we need it more than anyone ever has.

Habits of Relaxation and Activity

We aren't helpless victims of the stressful situations of modern life. The stress isn't *in* the situations, it's in us. We generate the effects of stress ourselves, however unwillingly. As Hans Selye puts it, "The crucial thing is not so much what happens to you, but the way you react to it."[184] The techniques grouped together under the term *meditation* provide a way to modify those reactions and deal with stress.

The medically relevant part of meditation consists of those effects which can be measured physiologically. It is clear that meditation can overcome the effects of stress, and can break the chain of stress-related events that can destroy tissue, consume nutrients at a destructive rate, impair the natural defenses against infection, and raise blood pressure. Although psychological measures are less precise than physiological ones, there are clear indications that the effects of meditation are desirable from a psychological point of view as well.

Benson's initial interest was in high blood pressure, and his

TM studies led to another possible tool for controlling it. But stimulating the relaxation response doesn't *cure* the problem, Benson is quick to point out. Once a diagnosis of high blood pressure is made, a patient is very probably committed to treatment for the rest of his life. However, *part* of the treatment, and in some cases all of it, could include practicing the relaxation response on a twice-daily basis. In many cases this has allowed the physician to decrease medication or to eliminate it altogether. (And here, Benson is careful to introduce a note of caution: If you are on medication for high blood pressure and begin meditation, check with your physician to see if he recommends adjusting the medication.)

High blood pressure is becoming increasingly widespread in industrialized countries because of the high level of stress. And it also stands in a vicious relationship with other diseases. The higher your blood pressure, the more prone you are to atherosclerosis, kidney disease, heart attack, and stroke.

Here is a good point to illustrate the difference between the Chinese approach to illness and the Western, and the way they are beginning to merge. We have become accustomed to dealing with each of the conditions mentioned in the preceding paragraph as a distinct disease; there are distinct medications, treatments, and in some cases surgical procedures, for each of them. Chinese medicine would view each of these conditions as a *symptom* of a more general problem of adjustment between the individual and the environment. One way to improve that adjustment is to learn to elicit the natural relaxation response that breaks the vicious chain of events that stress leads to. It is a little early to say that the role of the relaxation response in *preventing* high blood pressure has been established beyond doubt. This will require large, expensive, difficult investigations over a period of many years. However, in one recent study which contrasted people who practiced the technique with a control group of people who did not, those who regularly spent ten to twenty minutes twice a day eliciting the response had a lower incidence of high blood pressure.[128] The "carry-over effect"—the degree to which the relaxed state continues after the actual practice of the technique—seems to be as marked as the carry-over effects of stress itself.

It is the aspects of meditation that are not of direct medical relevance that will determine whether a person manages to incorporate it into his day-to-day habits. Most people need a framework of one sort or another in which to place this item of self-maintenance. The particular value of Benson's work is that it disentangles the measurable components of meditation practices from the complicated context of beliefs, goals, social commitments, and interpersonal relationships in which such techniques are typically taught.

Benson and his colleagues abstracted four basic elements from the particular details of many techniques. Each requires a mental device to focus the attention, a passive attitude toward the enterprise, a comfortable position, and a quiet environment. The many varieties of meditation that are being taught now all involve these basic ingredients, and as far as the physiological effects are concerned, one seems to be about as effective as another. The reasons for preferring one method have to do with matters of style and taste, and the embellishments. Don't let anyone tell you that there is only one way to do it, or only one program that can possibly work for you. That, like so much else in taking care of yourself, is a highly individual matter. The important thing is to find a program that is interesting and attractive enough that you will stay with it.

Now let's take the ingredients one at a time and look at the variations.

1. *The mental device.* The purpose of the device is to shift the attention away from "logical" and externally oriented thought. Some Zen meditators count their breaths; the TM

people and others of the yoga tradition use a nonsense word called a *mantra*, and you are asked to "think the sound" of the word; the Harvard group used the word "one"; and some religious meditators have used specific names for deities.

The use of visual imagery in place of a verbal device seems to be more common in hypnotic techniques, including Autogenic Training and the Mind Control technique associated with Jose Silva.

The device draws the conscious attention away from the details of the moment, and away from systematic and directed thought. Concepts are not engaged to discriminate elements in sensory experience. (This may be part of the reason why so much of Oriental philosophy views reality in terms of an undifferentiated unity.)

Sometimes the device to draw the attention consists of looking at an object or a candle flame. In this case, there is need for a protected and artificially controlled situation, because attention is easily distracted from the object by slight movements at the edges of the visual field.

2. *A passive attitude.* Passivity is difficult to achieve in the course of a hard-driving schedule. Thoughts and worries intrude. The impulse is to *suppress* thoughts, but this is not advised; it isn't just *letting things happen*, which is what it takes to get the appropriate biological response. The TM people compare thoughts to bubbles that come up from the lower depths of a liquid. They rise to the surface and break, but you don't get involved. Whatever happens during meditation just happens. Wolfgang Luthe, describing Autogenic Training, suggests a *casual* approach toward thoughts and toward the physiological effects one is seeking, advising that "Any goal-directed effort, active interest, or apprehensiveness must be avoided."[101]

3. *A relaxed position.* The posture generally recommended is upright but passive. No muscular effort should be required

to maintain it, and most systems recommend that legs, arms, hands, and feet not be crossed, since this increases the likelihood of decreased circulation or distracting sensory twitches. Zen meditators, on the other hand, use the lotus position to facilitate paying attention to the breathing, and other Japanese and Chinese disciplines use rhythmic, ritualized movements combined with a high level of concentration. The basic biological response can also be triggered during exercise or jogging, but the response can be elicited more quickly and more regularly, with less possibility of disruption, if the direct relaxation of muscles and body tone becomes a regular part of the program.

4. *A quiet environment.* The aim is simply to find a relatively private place, free from distraction, for fifteen or twenty minutes once or twice a day. Solitude isn't essential; once a regular habit of meditation is established, many people find it possible to meditate on a bus or train, or even sitting in a crowded auditorium or waiting room. In fact, people who are uncomfortable in planes often meditate through take-off rather than rely on tranquilizers.

The Transcendental Meditation people and some of the others argue convincingly that you are better off learning the technique from a person than you would be if you just read the instructions from a book. It is rather like learning to drive or learning to play a musical instrument. Most people need instruction, encouragement, support, and advice from an instructor in order to get the hang of it. If you decide to learn meditation from an individual who practices it, be as careful as you would be in choosing a driving instructor. If someone claims to have an approach to meditation that works, it should have worked for him.

If you decide to learn the technique through one of the organizations that incorporates it into a larger context, find out what to expect before you spend any tuition money. Almost every one of the popular packages has an "official" paperback or two describing the system, and that is as good a way as any to shop around. Most such groups offer free introductory lectures as well, so you can form some impressions of the people who practice the technique. Many weekend conferences on health, and some permanent programs in local hospitals, also teach the basic techniques.

The use of suggestion in the course of meditation or self-hypnosis has a long history, and it can be quite effective for some people. The method of Emile Coué, which enjoyed great popularity just after World War I, was essentially a self-hypnotic program wherein one repeated the slogan "Day by day, in every way, I'm getting better and better." A slogan or other means of planting positive suggestions along your daily path is also employed in Silva Mind Control and similar programs. Visual imagery to improve memory, deal with insomnia, cope with weight and smoking problems, keep resolutions, and otherwise improve yourself are incorporated into the basic relaxation technique.

Benson's four basic elements are not the only way to elicit the relaxation response. It has become clear that what is important to the response is not the specific element of being at rest, but rather breaking the chain of arousal that stimulates the hypothalamus to maintain a level of stress rather than the complementary level of relaxation. Articles have appeared recently about the emotional effects of jogging, suggesting that the basic relaxation response can be elicited while exercising. (Benson interprets the recent findings to indicate that the state of well-being begins after about four or five miles of jogging.) Some of the Oriental disciplines associated with the martial arts seem to elicit the basic response as part of a more complex pattern of responses, and such body-awareness programs as the Alexander Technique are directed toward combining bodily discipline and awareness with a level of concentration

and disengagement from daily concerns that somewhat resembles the basic relaxation response.

Incorporating one of these techniques into a daily routine or
"getting yourself out of the way," as Lester Fehmi describes it,
setting aside the tension and stress and eliciting an opposite,
restorative response, is a positive beginning to taking responsibility for your own well-being.

In any case, the important factor is habit. The difficulty in
using meditation only for first aid in times of stress is that the
habits don't sustain themselves that way. It is hardest to do at
the times when you need it most. Meditating regularly establishes the pattern, and once the relaxing habit is established, it
will be easier to stop in the middle of a high-pressure day and
break the pattern of stress. For that kind of immediate situation, it's cheaper and safer than tranquilizers.

Of course, it isn't *essential* to learn a meditative technique. If
your lifestyle includes a walk in the woods or a stroll along a
beach twice a day, you may well achieve some of the same
results.

Exercise can be an alternative to meditation and the other
relaxation techniques. Walking, jogging, calisthenics, or
swimming perhaps could be integrated in your daily routine.
Exercise maintains muscle tone and flexibility. Blood circulation improves, assuring the distribution of nutrients where they
are needed in the system. Exercising at least once a day to the
point of getting a little winded increases the strength of the
breathing muscles and insures good oxygenization of the
blood. Exercising to the point where the heartbeat perceptibly
speeds up strengthens the heart muscle. Several studies indicate that people who exercise tend to sleep better, worry less,
develop a positive self-image;[37] they are also likely to develop natural preferences for more nutritious foods because of
changes in metabolism and blood glucose levels, which affect
appetite and the desires for specific tastes.

Encounters and Disciplines: From Esalen to est

As you try to develop new attitudes toward yourself and your health, you are likely to find that your attitudes toward other people change, along with attitudes toward the institutions, goals and activities that occupy your time and attention. Many people feel that such changes in attitude are desirable, and popular psychological programs have been developed with attitudinal change as their goal.

In the late 1960s, about the same time the holistic movement was getting underway in medicine, a number of programs involving encounter groups and group therapy began to sprout, beginning at the Esalen Institute in the Big Sur region of California.

Esalen was the laboratory of the encounter-group movement. It provided a place for therapists to work out techniques to "open up" a personality through close and challenging contact with a group, and to help people develop a positive sense of themselves in relation to other people. The unaccustomed frankness and challenge of close personal contact with strangers in an intensive period of touching, talking, and doing things together constituted a sufficient break from daily roles and concerns that many people experienced changes in their long-range feelings that carried over into their everyday lives. Combined with massage, baths, exercises to enhance body awareness, and a general atmosphere of retreat from the artificial pressures of life, the encounters at Esalen produced dramatic changes in many people's thinking.

From that beginning, the encounter-group technique caught on with business, educational, and religious organizations. Many organizations arranged "T-groups" and "Encounter Weekends" for their management personnel in order to foster greater self-assertiveness and self-confidence. Encounters became a commercial fad for a time and took on something of the aspect of traveling shows. Well-known practitioners set up itineraries of prearranged groups, using Esalen techniques or their own variants. They set out to change the thinking and the lives of people in the course of intensive encounter sessions that lasted from a weekend to five or six days.

The difficulty with such artificial intensity was that many people found themselves severely disturbed by what happened in the encounters, and there was seldom an opportunity to follow up the initial challenge with long-range therapy or counseling. The practitioner moved on to the next stop, and the individual was left with a new awareness of conflicts he didn't know existed and no way to resolve them. The whistle-stop approach often did more harm than good.

Nevertheless, many people feel that they stand to gain from changing their points of view on themselves and their surroundings. The popularity of Oriental philosophy and the disciplines of Zen, yoga, and the martial arts testifies to the felt need for a fresh approach to life, a fresh way to sort out what is important from what is not. People hope to break old habits of thought by exposing themselves to alien points of view. Many of the Eastern disciplines can provide a framework within which to change exercise and eating habits, to develop a different sense of the body, and to develop habits and techniques that are involved in initiating the relaxation response.

A well-publicized commercial package that has gained nationwide appeal in recent years is est (Erhard Seminars Training), established by Werner Erhard. The initial "training session" consists of two full weekends of intense sessions, combining elements of Zen, yoga, Freudian technique, Dale Carnegie success training, encounter therapy, and "attack" therapy—all put together in such a way as to jar the participants into changing their attitudes toward themselves and their lives.

A recent book on est describes it as "not a religion, not

a therapy, not an academic course, and not a belief system . . . [but] theater—living theater, participatory theater, encounter theater."[138] The four-day training program has elements of all of these: religion, in that values are impressed upon the participants and a definite "congregational" community persists after the initiation; therapy, in that many facets of the training are directed toward shocking the participants into changing their attitudes by means of techniques borrowed freely from explicitly therapeutic contexts; and theater of the most method-ridden kind, because the instructors and the trainees are constantly engaged in acting out patently contrived situations on an intense emotional level.

The est training recalls those aspects of boot camp and fraternity hell week that formed such tight bonds among the young men of a generation or two ago. Although the transformation it claims is supposed to make one independent of the group, the graduates often form strong attachments to the organization and return to the group for reinforcement. At the guest seminars, where members are asked to bring new prospects for recruitment, it is apparent that many of them have not come to bring prospects at all, but to participate in the gathering of the congregation and to testify before the assemblage and experience the approval that such testimony brings.

Any measures you might take to change your outlook and your lifestyle are matters for individual decision. Finding out how other people think, how the Eastern philosophies approach matters of living, and how the thinking behind one of the meditative disciplines might fit into your life is easier now than it has ever been. In virtually every major city, one can learn yoga, Zen, or the martial arts, or participate in one of the programs that borrow freely from many sources.

For more directly medical matters, local programs and institutes for holistic health are beginning to develop all over the country. Some are more or less permanently established, or are connected with hospitals and other facilities, and have frequent courses, talks, informational services, and weekend workshops. Many of the programs are designed to inform people about new medical techniques, new means for self-care, or about ways of caring for family members who are seriously ill or dying. But most of the emphasis in the holistic workshops is on nutrition, stress relief, preventive health measures, exercise, dealing with transitions, and means for self-control and habit change—precisely the areas that each of us needs to take responsibility for, and where we might need individual advice.

Don't let the word *holistic* alone in someone's advertising draw you into a program. More and more, it will become a buzz-word. Look at the credentials of the people who run the program, and whose advice you will be paying for. Many people in the medical professions are becoming involved in holistic approaches to health and health care. It is no longer a matter of joining a counter-culture, and it isn't necessary to seek medical or psychological advice from people who are not qualified by training and experience to give it.

CHAPTER TEN

Nourishing a Stone-Age Body

The Arguments about Vitamin Supplements

The recent emphasis on our biological nature has led to a good deal of confusion and argument about nutrition. If our systems are essentially the same as those of our Stone-Age ancestors, if our organs, digestive systems, and nutrient needs haven't changed significantly in the past 10,000 years, how can we best nourish ourselves in twentieth-century America? Obviously we can't return to the lifestyle and eating habits of the hunter-gatherers. There are too many of us, for one thing, and we have changed the quality of human life far too drastically to revert now. Our sources of nourishment are not the lean animals and wild vegetables and fruits that provided human nourishment for the hundreds of thousands of years it took to establish the biological pattern. They are fat, well-fed, and genetically manipulated animals, produce that can be grown in large amounts and shipped over long distances, refined and concentrated foods, starches and sugars, and foods that have been treated in one way or another to keep them from spoiling. Moreover, the *amounts* of food we consume are significantly different from the amounts eaten by our primitive forebears; our lives are less active, our caloric needs are less. But our needs for specific nutrient substances are probably about the same.

The simplest forms of early life, organisms very much like bacteria, were able to put together all the compounds they needed from elemental raw materials found in mineral salts, nitrogen, carbon, and water. More developed species, including human beings, require more complex forms of nourishment; about fifty biochemical compounds and mineral elements are now recognized as essential for human life. So long as they are provided through our diet, the cells and tissues of the body can synthesize the other substances we need, and these number many thousands.

This result of biological evolution has in large measure shaped our social evolution. One of the reasons frequently given for the migration of human beings to the northern areas of the planet occurring so slowly is that the foods available in the winter did not contain sufficient ascorbic acid and other nutrients to sustain life.

The foods that established the biological needs of human nutrition were almost entirely fresh foods and that fact placed a limit on the variety that could be had at any given time and place. Today, we have a greater choice. Considering the enormous variety of foods available to us all year round, we should be able to maintain a diet that provides us with exactly what we need. But the appalling fact of the matter is that nobody knows exactly what an individual human being requires in the way of nutrients. (It follows that no prepackaged "formula" diet that you might buy in liquid or powder form can justify a claim that it provides everything you need.)

The concern with our genetic heritage has resulted in two main opposing lines of argument about nutrition: one group argues that, like our remote ancestors, we can get all the nutrients we need from foods if we choose them carefully; the other replies that under the conditions of modern life we need to supplement our foods, no matter how carefully they are chosen, with additional vitamins and minerals. Both sides recognize that our biochemical needs were established long before we became civilized, that the need for specific nutrients has not changed significantly since human beings stopped eating wild foods and started growing their own. Both sides agree that refined foods provide fuel in the form of calories without providing nourishment in the form of essential substances. But because the information about human needs is so spotty, there is disagreement about how to estimate those needs and how to be sure of meeting them.

The Food and Nutrition Board establishes a recommended daily allowance (RDA) of specific nutrients that can serve as a rule of thumb for making judgments about nourishment. But the Board cautions that the RDA should not be mistaken for a list of nutritional requirements. The information on which the RDA is based is severely limited because it is difficult and costly to test the nutritional needs of large numbers of people. The figures are therefore based on whatever the best available evidence is for a specific nutrient: studies with small groups of people, epidemiological studies of populations whose diet is deficient in a given nutrient, clinical studies of deficiency diseases, or studies with laboratory animals.

The RDA is confused by several factors. First, there is wide disagreement as to what an estimate of nutritional needs should be based on—the amounts of a nutrient necessary to prevent symptoms of a deficiency disease, or the amounts necessary to maintain a steady level of the nutrient in body tissues. The two figures are often quite different. Second, even if there were general agreement about which set of figures to use, neither can be specified for an entire population.

"Balance studies" measure the amount of a nutrient a person must consume in order to maintain a steady concentration in blood and tissues. The studies, difficult and expensive to perform, are carried out only on small groups for short periods. What they show is that the amount of any given nutrient needed to maintain a balance varies considerably from one person to the next, and that an individual's needs can change considerably as the circumstances of life change. For example, one study of nineteen healthy men showed that some needed four times as much calcium as others, and from two to seven times as much of the various amino acids.[182]

Some nutrients are not subject to this sort of study because they are impossible to measure in the human system. For fatty substances and vitamins, studies estimating human requirements are typically based on the amounts required to prevent the onset of detectable deficiency disease, although this means of estimation has obvious methodological and ethical limitations: the necessary experiments consist of generating disease in human subjects.

But neither kind of study is satisfactory because neither gives a clue to the amount of a nutrient that is necessary to maintain what is called *optimal nutrition*. According to Nevin Scrimshaw and Vernon Young of the Department of Nutrition and Food Science at MIT: "The overall nutrient balance might be achieved with a given intake of the nutrient being examined, but this does not prove that the tissues are functioning optimally and that health will be maintained."[144]

It is relatively easy to determine the kind of diet a cow or a sheep must have in order to maintain the best of health: by the quality of the fleece, or the milk, or, for that matter, the meat.

But it isn't so straightforward to make the same determination for human beings. Neither the best of health nor the amounts of nutrients required to maintain it are matters of general agreement.

There are enormous differences in the rate at which human beings use nutrients, and in the amounts of specific enzymes and proteins contained in individual systems. Pepsin and hydrochloric acid in the gastric juices can vary as much as 200-fold from one healthy adult to another.[182] Some of these differences are genetic, some are related to eating habits, amount and type of activity, or differences in body size. All of these, coupled with the variations in nutritional needs among people suffering from acute or chronic diseases make it impractical to estimate nutritional requirements for the entire population.[144]

The difficulties involved in finding a uniform set of nutritional recommendations lead some medical people virtually to ignore nutrition. At the other extreme, there are people both inside and outside the medical profession who think they have unlocked the secret of human nutrition, and who are ready to crusade for their own notions about special diets, special substances, huge amounts of this or that and none at all of something else. This leads to food fads. Both extremes, as usual, are wrong. However much nutritional needs may vary from one person to another, the *kinds* of nutrients needed by all human beings are the same.

Can we get all the vitamins, minerals, and other nutrients we need from the foods we eat without taking any supplements at all? Those who say that we can are, in general, the same people who accept the RDA as a reliable source of guidance about what it takes to nourish a given human being. They argue that vitamin supplements are unnecessary if we eat a great variety of foods. Medical students are generally taught that a healthy person eating a varied diet and balanced meals receives adequate amounts of vitamins. Some specialists in nutrition say, on the other hand, that most of our vegetables and fruits are raised on soil that has been too intensively farmed and is depleted in specific minerals, so that many of the foods we eat do not supply us with sufficient quantities of nutrients. Moreover, they argue, we don't eat sensibly all the time, and even if we did, food processing removes so many natural nutrients that diets must be augmented with vitamin supplements as insurance against subclinical deficiency diseases.[37,121]

Where those vitamins come from—the laboratory or the land—is also controversial. Both inexpensive synthetic vitamins and more expensive "natural" compounds are available. Once again, authorities disagree as to which way the choice should go. The difference between the two is simply that natural vitamins and minerals are refined from food sources like fish-liver oil in the case of vitamin A, or dessicated liver for some of the B vitamins and iron; synthetic vitamins come from a pharmaceutical laboratory. In the case of ascorbic acid, or vitamin C, the most popular natural source of the vitamin seems to be rose hips, to which some people are allergic. The arguments for using natural vitamins rest on the presence of trace substances that accompany the vitamin in its natural setting, and which might be important to its full effectiveness in the system.

However, the role of the trace substances that accompany identified vitamins and minerals in their natural settings isn't well understood. Clearly these can't be built into a vitamin pill synthetically, since in most cases, we don't know what the substances are, or which ones are needed to ensure the best use of the vitamin. According to the best evidence, the *primary* source of nutrition should be from the diet, not from a vitamin pill, natural *or* synthetic. Purifying natural substances in order to concentrate the vitamins probably does away with the natural setting of the vitamins among related substances, as animal studies indicate.

The findings are rather startling, in fact. A study was conducted to determine the link between adequate amounts of vitamins and the ability of the liver to produce a group of enzymes that inhibit the action of carcinogens. Laboratory animals were fed an artificial diet that included sufficient quantities of all *known* vitamins, minerals, and other nutrients in a highly purified form. The animals were unable to produce the important liver enzymes. When small amounts of alfalfa (one of the animals' natural foods) were added to the artificial diet, the enzyme production began almost immediately. Other fresh vegetables—cabbage, brussels sprouts, turnips, broccoli, cauliflower, dill, and celery—also enabled their systems to produce the anti-carcinogenic enzymes.[64]

In the argument about vitamin supplementation, it seems prudent to side with those who recommend at least a minimal supplement. Roger J. Williams, the biochemist who identified the B vitamin pantothenic acid, has done extensive research on how nutritional needs differ from one individual to another. He suggests a cautious "insurance" formula of vitamins, based on his judgment of "which nutrients are most likely to be deficient in the diets of the general population."[182] Williams says that "a supplement can be designed to augment, but not to substitute for, a balanced diet." Scrimshaw at MIT is inclined to think that a diet that is sufficiently varied and wisely chosen can make such supplementation unnecessary. The question then comes down to insuring yourself against the strength of your bad habits and the weakness of your good ones, and the strong possibility that much of the available food has lost nutrients before it gets to you or has been grown on depleted soil. If you choose foods carefully and you are confident of the quality of the foods available to you, it might be reasonable to forego the insurance Williams recommends. Otherwise, at least that much supplementation seems prudent.

There is an upper limit to prudent vitamin supplementation as well as a lower one. The arguments against indiscriminate vitamin supplementation generally focus on vitamins A and D, which are not excreted as quickly as other nutrients when there is an excess, and which can be toxic in excessively large doses. But Drs. Emanuel Cheraskin and W. M. Ringsdorf of the University of Alabama argue that the dosage at which vitamins A and D become toxic is so fantastically large that "You'd have to sit down and plan your own demise to take a damaging dosage of these nutrients."

Cheraskin and Ringsdorf recommend a slight excess of each known essential nutrient "as a hedge against malnutrition from primary or secondary dietary deficiencies." The special emphasis of their recommendations is on "brain-cell nutrients," which ensure proper neural function and provide protection against nutrient depletion caused by stress.[37]

It is generally recommended that any vitamin-mineral supplements be taken just before or during meals so that as many essential nutrients as possible will be present in the digestive tract at the same time, along with the setting of food substances that enhance their absorption and use.

In the accompanying table, the amounts of supplementary nutrients recommended by Williams for "nutritional insurance" are listed in the left-hand column, to establish the lower level of recommended supplementation. The next column lists the maximum amounts of the ranges of supplementary nutrients recommended by Cheraskin and Ringsdorf to guarantee optimal nutrition and the desired levels of brain-cell nutrients. The right-hand column shows the Recommended Daily Allowances, the conservative estimate of the amount of each nutrient required daily from all sources in order to avoid deficiency disease.

RANGE OF DAILY NUTRIENT INTAKE

Nutrient	Range of Recommended Supplementation	RDA
Vitamin A	7500 to 25000 units	5000 units
Ascorbic acid (vitamin C)	250 to 1500 mg	45 mg
Vitamin D	400 to 2500 units	400 units
Vitamin E	40 to 800 units	30 units
Vitamin K	2 — 2 mg	0.03 mg
Vitamin B1 (thiamine)	2 to 25 mg	1.5 mg
Vitamin B2 (riboflavin)	2 to 25 mg	1.8 mg
Vitamin B3 (niacin, niacinamide)	20 to 150 mg	20 mg
Vitamin B6	3 to 25 mg	2 mg
Vitamin B12	9 to 100 mcg	3 mcg
Pantothenic acid	15 to 200 mg	5–10 mg
Biotin	50 to 300 mcg	*
Folic acid	75 to 400 mcg	400 mcg
Choline	250 to 500 mg	*
Inositol	250 to 500 mg	*
PABA	30 to 50 mg	*
Rutin	200 — 200 mg	*
Bioflavinoids	50 to 300 mg	*
Calcium	250 to 1000 mg	800 mg
Phosphate	750 — 750 mg	800 mg
Magnesium	200 to 300 mg	350 mg
Iron	10 to 25 mg	10 mg
Zinc	2 to 20 mg	15 mg
Copper	0.5 to 2 mg	2 mg
Iodine	0.15 — 0.15 mg	0.14 mg
Manganese	5 to 20 mg	*
Molybdenum	0.1 — 0.1 mg	*
Chromium	1 — 1 mg	*
Selenium	0.02 — 0.02 mg	*
Cobalt	0.01 — 0.01 mg	*
Potassium	20 to 40 mg	2500 mg

Note: In addition, there are about twenty essential amino acids which cannot be synthesized but must be obtained from protein sources (meat and dairy products) and vegetable fats.

*No RDA has been established.

The use of huge amounts of single vitamins and minerals as a means of treating specific ailments is something that shouldn't be undertaken on the basis of one of those fragmentary reports in the press about some new bit of research. Most nutrients function properly in the system only when they are consumed in proportion with other nutrients. Overloading on a single vitamin alters the nutritional balance and can interfere with the utilization of other vitamins and minerals. Without expert advice, mega-vitamin consumption is not in general a good idea. There is one clear exception to this general principle, and it has been the subject of a good deal of controversy in the past decade: Ascorbic acid, known as vitamin C.

C: Don't Call It a Vitamin

Ascorbic acid, or vitamin C, appears throughout the medical literature. It is mentioned in books on cancer therapy, mental health, schizophrenia, the immune system, stress, burns and wounds, cells, and almost every human function.

Most of us first started paying attention to vitamin C at the time of Linus Pauling's *Vitamin C and the Common Cold* (1970). Pauling argued that about two grams of ascorbic acid daily would significantly reduce susceptibility to colds. Thus began the Vitamin C fad, and most medical practitioners dismissed Pauling's ideas as just that: another fad. A dozen or so studies have been carried out since then in the United States, England, and Scotland, and the most thorough one, in Toronto.[7] The conclusions are clear despite a few conflicting results:[82] Pauling is right. About two grams of vitamin C a day, for those who can tolerate it, substantially reduces the incidence and duration of colds.

But what about all those other ailments and functions? Why, one wonders, does ascorbic acid appear so often in the medical literature that has nothing to do with the common cold? Medical fads rarely have that kind of influence. Vitamin C, or ascorbic acid, begins to sound like some sort of super-substance, fit for every ill and needed in every function. And that, according to Dr. Irwin Stone, is exactly what it is.

It was Stone who first recommended vitamin C to Pauling in 1966, and he argues that it isn't a vitamin at all.[165] Vitamins are organic chemicals that we ordinarily get from foods, and they are essential in small amounts to our bodily functions. Other substances, such as glucose, dextrose, insulin, and proteins, are also essential, but they are needed in larger quantities than the vitamins are and can be produced in the body from raw materials in foods even though foods may not contain the substances. Stone argues that ascorbic acid and its related chemicals (the ascorbates) belong in this latter group.

Ascorbic acid is a relatively simple organic chemical, a carbohydrate closely related to the sugar glucose. Almost all plants and animals, from the simplest to the most complex, produce large quantities of ascorbic acid in their systems *from* glucose. But human beings, a few other primates, guinea pigs, and one species of fruit-eating bat in India cannot produce their own ascorbic acid. They must get it from the outside. A guinea pig deprived of ascorbic acid will die a horrible death from scurvy in two weeks.[165]

Ascorbic acid is needed for the proper functioning of almost every plant and animal. It is very active chemically and figures prominently in many of the important biochemical processes involved in the growth and maintenance of tissue. Beans, for example, contain very little ascorbic acid. But as soon as the beans start to sprout, the substance is present in large amounts. It is used in the formation of new plant tissues, and it is vital to the flexibility of the tissues and cells.

Ascorbic acid in the *human* system is used in a variety of ways:

1. To maintain homeostasis and resist stress. All the biochemical activity associated with stress requires ascorbic acid in

large amounts. In human beings stress, either emotional or physiological, depletes the amount of ascorbic acid in the blood and in the tissues most directly affected by the stress. In laboratory animals other than guinea pigs—that is, in those that can produce their own ascorbic acid—the substance is produced during stress. The more severe the stress, the more ascorbic acid is produced. If guinea pigs are given a diet low in ascorbic acid and then subjected to extreme stress, they die.

2. To aid in the production of collagen, one of the body's most important structural substances. Collagen is the cement that holds tissues and organs together and supports them. It keeps bones, arteries, and skin flexible, and it is the scar tissue that closes wounds. Without ascorbic acid we cannot produce collagen, and the tissue disease called scurvy occurs. With insufficient amounts of ascorbic acid, we still produce collagen, but it is weak, scarce, and faulty. A condition called subclinical scurvy results, which doesn't have the obvious and unpleasant symptoms of clinical scurvy but is nonetheless a dangerous weakening of bodily tissue.

3. As a catalyst in metabolism. Ascorbic acid speeds the action of digestive enzymes, as well as other chemical activities that are important to the maintenance of proper body chemistry. It activates insulin, which we need to metabolize sugar. Stone sees good evidence for the hypothesis that maintaining an optimal level of ascorbic acid may help to prevent diabetes.

4. As an aid in the function of the nervous system and brain. Here the connections are not well understood. Studies show that the level of ascorbic acid in the bodies of schizophrenic patients is abnormally low; that they metabolize the substance ten times as fast as nonschizophrenics. Large doses of ascorbic acid administered to schizophrenic patients produced uniformly marked improvement.[174] Other studies

show that the substance is essential to the biochemistry of both the brain and the nervous system.

5. As a detoxicant. A number or surprising European studies show that ascorbic acid enhances our ability to throw off poisons, that it can be used as an antidote in lead poisoning and that it prevents kidney damage in arsenic poisoning.[107] Most likely it speeds up the natural defenses against poisons by its catalytic effect on our biochemistry. In addition, it is depleted rapidly in the recovery from carbon dioxide poisoning, and it is well known that smoking also depletes it. Stone calls the depletion resulting from this detoxicant use of ascorbic acid "smoker's scurvy." Smokers who do not consume sufficient quantities of ascorbic acid develop the early signs of "subclinical" scurvy, because the substance is consumed in the system's attempts to deal with the toxins in tobacco smoke. One cigarette depletes the system of about 25 milligrams.

Some of the more frightening toxins are the nitrites found in smoked meats and fish, and even in beer. Upon digestion, they generate *nitrosamines,* which are powerful carcinogens. A 1972 University of Nebraska study showed that if ascorbic acid is present when nitrites are introduced into the stomach, the cancer-causing nitrosamines do not form.

6. To aid the immune system in fighting infection and cancer. Ascorbic acid controls and maintains *phagocytosis,* the action of the white blood cells in the immune system. If the ascorbic acid level in the blood is low, white blood cells will not so readily attack, ingest, and destroy bacteria and other unwelcome bits of material, including abnormal cells generated within the body itself. The importance of ascorbic acid in the action of the immune system has been known since 1943; and in 1969 a study by the National Cancer Institute showed that ascorbic acid is lethal to some cancer cells and harmless to normal tissue. But only recently have studies been carried out

with cancer patients to determine how ascorbic acid stimulation of the immune system might affect the disease. The results, with rather high doses, have been encouraging.[19]

7. As a bactericide, viricide, and antiseptic. Maintaining a high level of ascorbic acid in the blood (by taking about 7,000 milligrams a day) kills bacteria, or stops their growth, independent of the action of the immune system. In many cases of viral infection, including poliomyelitis, herpes, and hepatitis, similar effects have been noted.[165]

That's an impressive list of functions for one relatively simple organic chemical. Why can almost every other form of life on this planet produce its own ascorbic acid, when human beings cannot? As Irwin Stone tells it, one of our primate ancestors, millions of years ago, underwent a genetic mutation that destroyed his ability to produce the enzyme L-gulonolactone oxidase, one of four enzymes needed to convert glucose into ascorbic acid. The other three enzymes remained and continued the attempt to make ascorbic acid, but without that fourth enzyme, the last step in the process couldn't be completed.

If an animal species loses the ability to carry out an important part of the biochemical activity that sustains life, it ordinarily dies out. But why didn't the primates become extinct? For the same reason that the guinea pigs and the Indian bats didn't. They ate a diet that was very high in ascorbic acid. Primates and guinea pigs live on fresh green plants, the bats on fruits, all of which supply significant amounts of ready-made ascorbic acid. So long as there is a minimal level of ascorbic acid in the system, the animals live at least long enough to reproduce.

As human beings migrated around the world, they were able to maintain the small amount of ascorbic acid needed for survival by adjustments in their diet. That's part of the reason for some of the dietary oddities in specific groups. Why do Eskimos eat raw fish and meat? It turns out that cooking meat and fish reduces the ascorbic acid content. Since vegetables are not readily available in the far north, raw fish and raw meat are the best sources of the substance. Somewhere, thousands of years back when they first settled in the north, the Eskimos learned that a diet of raw fish and meat would sustain life, while a diet of the same items cooked would not.

According to Stone, our inability to produce ascorbic acid amounts to a hereditary disorder, a genetic disease that requires us to take special measures throughout our lives. It is another one of those items of evolutionary fitness that was well taken care of in the lifestyles of our Stone Age ancestors, but that in modern life requires some behavioral adjustment. Pauling estimates that our ancestors ate raw fruits, vegetables and greens that totaled about 2,500 calories per day. This would supply about 2,300 milligrams of ascorbic acid, enough to meet the system's needs under ordinary circumstances. (That's about 51 times the amount officially recommended on the government nutrition charts.) Since our lifestyles are different from those of our ancestors, we need to correct the deficiency with a dietary supplement, according to Stone, Pauling, and a growing list of researchers.

By estimating the amounts of ascorbic acid produced naturally in the systems of other mammals, Stone calculates that the average adult requires between two and four grams of ascorbic acid per day under conditions of little or no stress. When there is stress, however, the amount manufactured by other mammals is multiplied several times, since the consumption of ascorbic acid increases dramatically. Adults subject to stress are estimated on this basis to need as much as 15 grams per day.

The distinctly biological arguments offered by Stone and Pauling in favor of dietary supplementation with ascorbic acid have convinced many people both inside and outside the medical profession. Long-range studies of the effects of large amounts of synthetic ascorbic acid have not been completed, however, and some medical people caution that kidney problems might arise from excessive supplementation. The substance occurs naturally in every form of animal and plant life, not just in citrus fruits; diets which include large amounts of fresh fruits and vegetables will require less supplementation to reach Stone's figure of two to four grams.

Diet, Stress, and the "Responses"

Like many people, I have always thought of nutrients primarily in terms of substance—the "building blocks" of tissue, bone, and muscle. Activity, exercise, the things I *do,* have always seemed to be connected more with fuel, calories burned up in the system to produce energy. I was dead wrong. Every activity, conscious and unconscious, requires specific vitamins and other nutrients.

The immune response, for example, including the production of antibodies and lymphocytes, as well as the elements of cell-mediated immunity, is severely limited when there is a vitamin deficiency, particularly vitamin A. And about 25 percent of those tested in a United States National Nutrition Survey showed low serum levels of vitamin A.[134] Deficiencies in vitamin E, the B complex, dietary proteins, ascorbic acid, iron, and potassium have all been shown in animal studies to inhibit cell-mediated immunity, which figures in both resistance to infection and the weeding out of cancer cells.[34]

At the same time, there is a danger from over-nutrition, especially when the diet is high in fats and calories. Studies with overfed dogs indicate that obesity and a high-calorie maintenance diet severely suppress the resistance to virus infections.[115] This is partly because of a relationship between obesity and substances related to immune response, and partly because fatty tissue provides a particularly hospitable place for viruses to multiply. A similar connection may also exist between obesity and a tendency toward cancer, a suspicion arising from epidemiological figures comparing the incidence of the disease in populations consuming differing amounts of fat. Dr. Elizabeth M. Whelan, a research associate at the Harvard School of Public Health, writes, "I can't explain the major world differences in breast cancer, for instance, without bringing in high fat, over-nutrition.[126] Both refined carbohydrates like sugar and alcohol, and saturated fats like those found in beef and pork, have been identified as *susceptibility agents.* An over-supply of them increases the likelihood of disease.[37]

What you require nutritionally changes as your activities change and as you age. It varies with climate, emotional tension, stress, the amount of sexual activity, the amount of exercise, and the day-to-day demands you put on your energies. Moreover, individual needs vary for genetic reasons, and because the forms in which we ingest specific nutrients cause variation in the way we absorb them. It is easier, for example, to absorb iron from meat than from vegetable sources.[144]

The presence or absence of one nutrient often affects the utilization of another. Proteins are essential for the transport of vitamin A in the system. If the diet is deficient in protein, the vitamin remains stored in the liver and cannot be used, so a deficiency disease can develop even when the vitamin A intake *by itself* is sufficient.

Stress depletes the supply of specific nutrients in the system, and it does so quite rapidly in the case of the B vitamins, ascorbic acid, vitamin E, and the minerals zinc and copper. One natural response can weaken another: When nutrients are depleted because of the stress response, they become unavailable for the action of the immune response, and we are more subject to infectious disease. In addition, stress increases the activity in neurons containing the neurotransmitters norepinephrine and serotonin in the higher parts of the brain. Since certain amounts of these substances are metabolized each time they function in a neural synapse, they must be constantly replenished by the system. That means that the chemical precursors of neural chemicals must be supplied in greater amounts by the diet.

Trauma, anxiety, fear, and other causes of stress have a pronounced effect on protein requirements. Stress increases the rate of the breakdown of muscle protein into amino acids, which are transported to the liver to be converted into glucose, in order to support a burst of energy. Some of these amino acids are required for the synthesis of neural chemicals. Recovery from stress entails replacing the protein and amino acids so that both muscle tissue and neural chemicals are not left depleted.

Beyond the specifically identified physiological responses, emotional states and emotional problems have been linked to minor vitamin deficiencies, which are not at all rare among well-fed Americans. Even a mild deficiency in niacin, for example, can be linked to insomnia, nervousness, irritability, and depression, and in severe cases to hallucination. These problems can be improved by supplementation of the vitamin. But a recent survey of the diets of male doctors in this country showed that one out of eight did not receive even the minimal amount of niacin called for in the Recommended Daily Allowance.[37]

A major part of the connection between diet and emotional states has to do with the need to supply the system with the precursors of the neurotransmitters and neuroregulators, which are necessary for the functioning of the brain and the nervous system. Adequate neural function depends on the neural chemicals being present in sufficient supply. The old tales about certain diets providing "brain food" had something to them after all. Some researchers believe that most mental illness is linked to nutritional deficiencies in the B vitamins, ascorbic acid, the amino acids (especially lysine, threonine, and the neurotransmitter-precursor tryptophan), choline, and inositol.[37,181] While some doubt remains that such deficiencies are a major cause of emotional problems on a nationwide basis, the matter cannot be determined strictly. There is *no* doubt, however, that maintaining a supply of nutrients that is both adequate and, perhaps more important, that is in balance, is essential to proper brain function. That, in turn, is intimately associated with the prevention of disease and the recuperation from disease and injury.

Informed Judgments about Food and Health

There is no way that this book or any other book can set down a program of healthy habits that will be appropriate for everyone. The point has emerged in every area of human health that we have covered: the individual differences among people are too great for any one program to be right for all of us. What *can* be set down is a basis for making some sound judgments about taking care of yourself in your own situation, and for developing habits of daily living that meet your personal needs. Forming such habits is a matter of judgment and determination, and an important part of assuming full responsibility for your own state of health and well-being. Everyone has to make such individual judgments, even the people who are directly involved in medical research and health care.

The *Medical Tribune* recently asked fourteen prominent experts—researchers, officers of research organizations, and medical school professors—how they personally try to safeguard themselves against cancer. Their answers revealed the extent to which such safeguards are a highly personal matter, and the extent to which personal judgments differ even among the best-informed professionals.[126] The query didn't ask for a full description of lifestyle, but only for those personal habits that are specifically directed toward avoiding cancer. Two of the medical experts said that their only anti-cancer measure was to avoid smoking and to avoid people who smoke. The remaining twelve mentioned diet and nutrition: seven avoid fats, three avoid food additives and preservatives, three either avoid alcohol altogether or have cut down on drinking, and two avoid sugar.

Among the positive steps taken to avoid cancer, six of the twelve mentioned vitamins, and five of those made particular mention of vitamin C. Four use an "insurance formula" of vitamins and minerals. Other specific nutrients mentioned were vitamins A, E, the B complex, B6, folic acid, calcium, and magnesium.

In planning meals, five mentioned high fiber and low-fat foods, and three spoke of "wholesome" foods or fresh vegetables. Three mentioned eating *less* food in order to keep weight down, and others said that they eat less meat than they used to. Other specific anti-cancer strategies mentioned were exercise and regular medical examinations, and in the case of one person with light coloring and sensitive skin, staying out of the sun.

The overall list of items that one or more of the experts consider relevant to cancer prevention is nearly identical to the list of items linked to high blood pressure and heart disease. In fact, the risk factors involved in all the "diseases of civilization" are similar: pollutants, smoking, inadequate nutrition and physical activity, stress, and infrequent medical examinations and lack of medical care. The differences among the habits of the fourteen experts emphasize that there is more than one reasonable interpretation of the research linking personal habit with disease risk, and that individual differences require individual adjustments of lifestyle. At the same time, the similarities among the responses provide some guidance—not about how to adapt your own habits perhaps, but about how to make decisions about adapting them. Your life situation is probably quite different from that of any one of those fourteen experts. Your own combination of inherited characteristics, household matters, employment, age, and personal history will no doubt make your own "best adaptation" somewhat different from any of theirs.

But the questions you need to answer for yourself are the same ones the experts had to answer. First, what should you avoid? Known carcinogens, surely. You cannot avoid them entirely, but as the high-risk carcinogens like asbestos and vinyl chloride are identified, they can be eliminated from the environment, and the lower-risk carcinogens can be kept to a minimum. The control of carcinogenic industrial pollutants, however, is more a matter of public policy than of individual action, except in the sense that we as vocal, informed voters can influence that policy.

In the area of food the panel of cancer experts specifically avoid additives, preservatives, and excessive amounts of refined carbohydrates. Forming constructive habits concerning food and nutrition is the first step in ensuring that you will get sufficient amounts of essential nutrients, while minimizing your consumption of the things that are best avoided.

As uneasy as it makes one feel to realize that unavoidable elements in human life, including natural factors like sunlight, can cause the mutation of cells, remember that one single mutant cell is *not* cancer. The aim must be to avoid the combinations of circumstances that allow mutant cells to develop into cancerous growths That means maintaining a high level of resistance as well as avoiding known carcinogens.

Smoking presents a special problem. It is probable that everyone who could stop easily has already done so. What remain are the hard-core cases. Your personal smoking habit, if you have one, is just that: yours *personally*. Programs and anti-smoking measures are effective for some but not for others; however, the habit can be tackled in many different ways. Hospitals and medical associations, such as those for cancer and heart disease, provide smoking clinics. Hospital psychologists who employ hypnosis with cancer patients are often available to private patients with smoking problems. Many people find it easier to stop smoking once they have begun taking steps to deal with stress through meditation or one of the other ways of eliciting the relaxation response. People who exercise regularly tend to smoke less. Physicians at some hospitals use various forms of acupuncture to help people break the habit. In addition, commercial stop-smoking organizations offer specific programs. The only sensible thing to do if you are one of the hard-core cases is to keep trying until you succeed in stopping altogether.

Establishing a Healthful Diet

One thing nutritionists all seem to agree on is the need for diversity in the diet. They emphasize that there is no complete list of human dietary needs, that the exact quantities required of the known essential substances cannot be specified for every individual, and that each individual's needs vary considerably in the natural course of events as activity, stress, age, the state of health, and the seasons of the year change. The one way to assure adequate nutrition under those circumstances is to eat a broad variety of foods. No one food can provide all the nutrients you need, and no combination of foods, repeated over and over on a daily or weekly basis, will do the job either. A good selection of fruits, vegetables, meats, fish, dairy products, and grain foods, with plenty of variety within each of those groups, is available year round and food choices are best if they take advantage of that happy fact.

There is a less pleasant reason for keeping your diet varied: the moving target argument. Dr. Gary Flamm, a toxicologist in the FDA's Bureau of Foods, told an interviewer, "My philosophy is to spread the risk. If I ate one thing (in excess) I'd be in trouble."[15] Because we don't yet have full information concerning the effects of additives, preservatives, insecticides and industrial chemicals that find their way into the food supply and may tend to concentrate in one plant or animal, it is simply not prudent to concentrate your diet on one single food. Moreover, dangerous or disagreeable substances occur naturally in tiny quantities in some foods. For example, one natural fungus, a precursor of aflatoxin, a substance known to promote cell mutation, forms on peanuts and whole grains in storage. However, in a varied diet the quantities likely to be eaten are almost infinitesimal. But if you were to eat these foods to the exclusion of others, as some fad diets suggest, those tiny quantities of natural carcinogens could add up sufficiently to constitute a risk.

Most nutritionists stress the advantages of fresh foods over processed and preserved foods. In general, preserved foods are depleted in nutrients to some degree when compared with fresh local products, and they should be used only when fresh foods are out of season. On the other hand, Dr. Nevin Scrimshaw, head of the Department of Food and Nutrition Science at MIT, cautions that out-of-season fresh vegetables that have been shipped long distances or stored for long periods lose nutrients too, so there is no nutritional reason to prefer them over canned or frozen vegetables.

There is also general agreement that highly refined and processed foods should be kept to a minimum; processing and pre-cooking decreases nutritive value. Bleached flour is widely denounced as nutritionally worthless, even when it is "enriched." The bleaching process removes more than twenty vitamins, minerals, and amino acids; the "enrichment" restores only four of these.[37] Sugar and alcohol supply calories but not nutrients, and heavy consumption of either can lead to the over-production of fat. Evidence shows that sugar also lowers the *phagocytic index,* a measure of the effectiveness of the immune response.[19]

Weight loss is made more difficult because it is easy with refined foods to overeat. Fad diets that concentrate on a narrow range of foods are generally considered to be nutritionally limited and potentially dangerous. There is only one good way to lose weight, it seems, and that is to eat less, while at the same time maintaining a varied diet. Also, whole-grain unrefined foods tend to be more filling as well as more nourishing. Many people who try limited-variety diets suffer mild emotional disturbance after the first week. Cheraskin and Ringsdorf's summary of the research connecting nutrition and neural chemistry shows that even limiting the variety of nutrients can lead to severe emotional problems, by depleting the system's supply of those substances they identify as "brain nutrients." Even a reducing diet should be balanced and varied.

Many specific foods and vitamins have been claimed to have "anti-cancer" properties, inhibiting the development of abnormal cells and in some cases even curing the disease. Anti-cancer claims have been made for specific vegetables, notably asparagus,[19] and those found to encourage the production of anti-carcinogenic liver enzymes in the animal experiments described earlier: broccoli, cauliflower, cabbage, brussels sprouts, turnips, alfalfa, dill, and celery. Most of the claims are based on anecdotal records of individual experience, with no systematic clinical testing to back them up, partly because funds have not been available, and partly because there is not sufficient preliminary evidence to justify a major research effort.

The general guidance that has emerged from nutrition research can be summarized for the main groups of foods.

Fiber

In general, whole-grain foods, bran, and fiber have a good deal to recommend them besides the nutrients they contain because of their overall effect on the digestion, speeding up the "transit time" between eating and elimination and thus reducing the possibility that wastes will stagnate in the system and possibly generate carcinogens. In addition, fiber from grain and vegetable sources binds with cholesterol and bile salts in the intestines, aiding in their elimination. Studies carried out at the U.S. Department of Agriculture's Human Nutrition Laboratory indicated that cereal fiber reduces the levels of serum cholesterol and low-density lipoproteins in the blood.[27] One way to increase variety in the diet and to incorporate more natural fiber is of course to experiment with unfamiliar foods. Some whole-grain foods available in natural foods stores seem at first to be unappetizing, but they should provide sufficient choice for a good variety of fiber-rich foods.

Vegetables

The nutritionists' advice concerning vegetables comes down to a simple set of general principles: Vary vegetables as much as possible; take advantage of local fresh vegetables in season. For maximum vitamin content, raw vegetables are in general better than cooked; undercooked and crunchy vegetables are better than overcooked and soggy ones; steaming or stir-frying is better than boiling.

Meats and Other Protein Sources

Several of the medical experts surveyed about anti-cancer measures specifically stated that they avoid fatty meats, and eat less meat than they used to. Epidemiological studies show that beef in particular should not be consumed in excess. But beef is nourishing and high in protein, and it is a staple in the American diet. There is no reason to eliminate any kind of nourishing food altogether, although there is very good reason to reduce the consumption of beef. Fatty meats should be kept to a minimum, according to most nutritionists, and leaner meats such as chicken and fish should play a larger role in the diet, along with eggs, cheese, and other dairy products.

Fats and Oils

Oils low in saturated fats and high in polyunsaturates have been recommended for a long time as a means for controlling serum cholesterol. While many authorities now hold that diet does not play a large role in producing cholesterol in the blood-stream (cholesterol is produced in the body regardless of the diet), increasing the proportion of polyunsaturates in the diet aids in the metabolism of saturated fats. Vegetable oils that are hydrogenated to make them the consistency of butter are not particularly good for this purpose; The liquid oils have the polyunsaturated advantage, although olive oil is very high in saturated fats. Of the inexpensive oils, corn oil has the most unsaturated fats; safflower oil, which is even better, is available in some places at comparable prices. Rather than eliminate butter and olive oil altogether, they can be mixed with unsaturated vegetable oils. In cooking, for example, or for garlic butter, one part butter to two or three parts corn oil, or even a half-and-half mixture, improves the nutritional situation without eliminating favorite flavors. One part olive oil to four to ten parts of less saturated oils is ideal for salad dressing.

Such measures as these constitute sensible adjustments in eating habits; they don't turn the kitchen into a clinical laboratory or take all the joy out of eating good food.

From a nutritional point of view, taking responsibility for your own health entails understanding both the biological needs common to all human beings, which determine the *kinds* of nutrients you require, and the needs that arise out of your individual way of life, which determine the *amounts* of nutrients you require. It comes down to a matter of personal hygiene, to establishing a set of sensible eating habits that, along with sensible habits of exercise, relaxation, and self-maintenance, will minimize the risk of disease, maximize your ability to cope with problems that do arise, and increase the likelihood of your maintaining what is for you, individually, the best of health.

CHAPTER ELEVEN

The Impact of Holism

Why Holism Makes Sense Now

Taken by itself, any one of the medical developments described in this book would be an oddity. Taken together, and unified by the holistic conception of what it is to be a person, they constitute a picture of a fresh approach to health research and health care. It is a mistake to associate holism with any single medical discovery or technique, or even with a particular lifestyle or system of health care. Holism is a way of thinking about human beings, a way of trying to come to a better understanding of our own nature and the influences on our health and well-being. This way of thinking is becoming widespread among people in the medical and research professions, and among people like you and me—the consumers of medical care.

When a new idea catches on, it catches on for a reason. The intellectual and scientific settings have to be right. The technology has to be available to test the consequences of the new conception and to apply it in useful ways. There has to be a felt need for change, and the established way of approaching problems has to be under serious challenges in the form of problems it cannot deal with. If holism is taking hold in medicine and psychology as I have been suggesting, with the power of an idea whose time has truly come, then we should be able to see a more general change in attitudes that constitutes the larger setting in which this particular change is taking place. And we can. Apart from the distinctly scientific considerations discussed earlier, this is a time of general reappraisal of the way we live our lives and the way we relate to the rest of the world. Americans are taking a cold, hard, realistic look at the way we consume energy and other resources, at the ratio between the energy involved in doing a task and the rewards obtained when the task is done. Changing circumstances and needs are causing us to think again about how and where we travel, how we heat our homes, how we utilize space, the ways we use electric power, and the products we consume. Political and economic considerations as well as ecological ones have made people concerned about the possible over-uses and abuses of technology, which is often employed simply because it is possible. This is as true in manufacturing, business, and transportation as it is in the area of health care. And at the same time, many of us are having second thoughts about how and where we apply our own human energy and resources.

We need to pay attention to different things than we have paid attention to in the past when planning our lives, and we know it. We feel the need to look at ourselves in relation to the world in a new way. The increasing interest in the thinking and techniques of other times and other cultures indicates a need to explore alternative approaches to human problems. This need is felt as much within the sciences and the other formal disciplines as it is among the public at large.

The three general principles that I used earlier to characterize holism are not new to Western thought. They have appeared from time to time in the literature of medicine, biology, and psychology for fifty years or more, and each of them has been held in the past as part of a larger system of thought. It seems clear that they are finding an influential place now in the mainstream of the human sciences, as well as in the thinking of people outside the medical professions. And they are not as easy and obvious as they seem to be.

Take the first of the three principles: that a human being is one thing, not two; that the mind and the body cannot meaningfully be distinguished. This is a particularly difficult point for many of us who grew up in the Western tradition. Our thinking about ourselves has been structured for over three hundred years by the sharp distinction between the mental and the physical that was spelled out explicitly by Descartes. The "mind-body problem" has occupied the attention of psychologists and philosophers throughout the whole period in which high technology and theory have developed in the West. The "body" side of the problem posed no great difficulty so long as the human body could be regarded as part of the complex machine of nature. But the line between the mental and the physical never came into sharp focus, and the "mind" part of the problem has been troublesome enough to raise questions about whether or not there ever could be a genuine science of human psychology. Over the centuries, there have been two main lines of reasoning about that group of events in human experience that are classed as mental. On the one hand, many people have agreed with Descartes that mental events are of a different kind than physical events, that they are occult—hidden—and essentially private, and that they cannot therefore be subjected to systematic, objective study in the way that physical events can. This is good old-fashioned dualism. People in this corner agreed with Descartes that the mind was a separate entity from the body, and that any discussion of an individual's mental life was best left to theologians and mystics, and perhaps to an occasional psychoanalyst. But it was surely not the province of hard scientists.

On the other hand, many people in the sciences came to regard all talk of mental events as spurious, a fiction of language. If all of nature is governed by strict mechanical laws, they argued, then human nature must be governed by those laws too. The human organism must differ from animals, and even from machines, *only* in its complexity; and it is that complexity that has led us to suppose, erroneously, that there is some addtional element, called "mind," that enters into human experience. This is a materialist view, and it carries with it a commitment to *reduce* the vocabulary for describing human beings by reformulating all statements about a person's thoughts, sensations, emotions, and intentions as statements about bodily states and observable behavior. If the reduction had ever been carried out successfully, it would have brought all talk about mental events within the scope of strict physical laws, and would eventually have allowed us to predict and to manipulate human activity in a deterministic way.

The reductivist argument was extremely appealing in the setting of Newtonian science, and it still has many adherents in both psychology and the physical sciences. There is a strong and widely held article of faith that a full description of all human functions and activities can eventually be given in purely mechanistic terms. But it should be recognized by both the adherents and the opponents of this claim that it does involve an article of faith. The claim has been taken seriously for more than sixty years now, and nobody has yet come anywhere close to making good on it. There is no good reason to suppose that anyone will ever make good on the reductivist claim, apart from the doctrine that every natural event can eventually be understood in mechanical terms. The burden of proof must now rest with the strict behaviorists and other reductivists if we are to take that claim seriously any longer. Otherwise, the demand for reduction must be viewed as a peculiar outgrowth of the attempt to study human beings by means of a prior study of mechanical systems, of trying to do human psychology as ultimately an outgrowth of nineteenth century physics.

Holism, as a third alternative to dualism and reductionism, is relatively new in the literature of Western science and philosophy. The arguments between dualists and reductivists over the decades have made it clear that neither view provides a satisfactory foundation for a science which purports to explain both human activity and human experience—the kind of science that any ultimately successful approach to medicine and psychology must rest on. The critical dialogue about the concept of a person in the dominant British-American tradition of philosophical psychology began in earnest with Peter Strawson's attempt to spell out the consequences of treating the person as a functional unit to which one can ascribe both states of consciousness and bodily characteristics. Strawson and his successors have argued that these two sets of "predicates" are irreducible—that one set cannot be abandoned in favor of the other without loss of meaning—but that they should not be understood as designating the characteristics of two separate entities. The argument puts holism at odds with both the reductivists and the dualists.

Thus, as Joseph Margolis argues, moving your hand in such a way as to volunteer for a job cannot be understood in purely physical terms, or as a simple matter of response to a stimulus.[106] It is *correct* to describe the action in terms of neural and muscular activity, but you can't tell the whole story in those terms. It is also correct to describe it as a bit of behavior in response to the complex stimulus of the call for volunteers, but you can't tell the whole story in those terms either. To describe the action fully and understand its causes and consequences, we have to call on those properties that are peculiar to persons: the cultural context where conventional uses of language and gestures are well understood, the individual context of beliefs, desires, and expectations that has been shaped by the cultural setting, the capabilities and limitations that are part of human nature, and, finally, the intention which led you to raise your hand and volunteer in the first place. A person has biological properties as well as culturally emergent properties; linguistic habits and capacities as well as biochemical habits and capacities; physical properties as well as intentions and expectations. But all of these are properties of a single entity, and they are interrelated.

Depression, for example, can be described accurately as a particular kind of felt emotion, or as a subtle set of bodily sensations, or as a physico-chemical state of the nervous system. The descriptions are all of the same range of events, but they employ different vocabularies and they are not in any sense equivalent. From a medical point of view, the interrelations among all these distinct modes of description have assumed a new importance, because each provides an angle of attack on the problem of depression in human experience. To identify depressed states, *and* discuss how they are triggered, *and* discuss their consequences and causes, we need to have *every* angle of approach open for serious study.

This first principle of holism has had considerable impact on the recent medical concern about our adaptation to modern life. It means that we cannot adequately understand our individual responses to the environment without taking into consideration the ways that we have learned to interpret sensory information and respond to it. It means that the fight-or-flight response, for example, with all its implications for our states of health, can only be understood, modified and manipulated by understanding the individual's intentions, desires and expectations, as well as the perceptual context in which certain situations are identified as threatening and others are not. The division between the mental and the physical is not one that we find in human nature; it is a distinction that we have learned to make, and it has ceased to be useful in describing many medically relevant areas of human experience.

The second major principle of holism is that a person is a tightly organized biological unit, not a set of discrete mechanisms that just happen to be wired together. The scientific side of our culture has been occupied for a long time with analysis, with isolating the objects it studies and determining what makes them tick individually in their "pure state." But the intellectual style throughout our culture is gradually turning from analysis to synthesis, to examining objects in their natural setting, and asking how specific items fit in with the rest of the world. The organs of the human system don't exist in a pure and isolated state. Their structure and nature, their functions and malfunctions, must be understood within the overall context of the whole living organism. The holistic motto that medicine must treat the whole person, not just the damaged parts, has been illustrated by the many medical developments described in the preceding chapters. Whether we are seeking cures for disease or more generally trying to determine what it takes to maintain an optimum state of health, it is the whole organism that must be considered. The efficient action of the immune system, for example, cannot be localized to those areas of the brain where the response is triggered, or to those areas of the digestive system and the bloodstream where the nutrients essential to the response are supplied, or even to the particular area where the response may be in action to deal with infection or abnormal cells. We can no longer suppose that the brain and the nervous system are somehow separable from the rest of the organism, and we can no longer describe our own states in purely local terms, given the complexity of any human response to changes in our surroundings. This is true of those human characteristics traditionally regarded as psychological, as well as those which have been regarded as physiological.

Anxiety, for example, is no more "all in the mind" than ulcers are all in the duodenum. The biochemical states which are associated with felt anxiety involve the entire system, as the effectiveness of tranquilizers and nutritional therapy for chronic anxiety demonstrate. Ulcers and heart ailments have their root causes in biochemical states and habitual patterns of emotional arousal that cannot meaningfully be localized. And as we have seen, cancer, wherever it manifests itself, has come to be regarded as a disease of the entire organism.

Holistic thinking should not be confused with the kind of careless "global" outlook that insists on the relevance of everything in the world to everything else in the world. You can generate as much patent nonsense in that direction as you can by supposing that each natural object can be understood apart from its context. Connections need to be traced and demonstrated. But the emerging connections linking diet with behavior and emotion, and all of these with natural defenses against disease, for example, suggest strongly that both the prevention and the treatment of disease must be approached with the whole human system in mind.

Finally, the third holistic principle demands that we see ourselves as part of the world around us. Like the other two principles, this one seems obvious and unobjectionable on the face of it, until you reflect on the fact that we in the West have characteristically considered ourselves to be "above" our natural environment and separate from it. As technology developed and civilization became more complex, we tended to ignore the ecosystem and our relationship to it. The generally sensible movement in favor of the ecology that has taken hold in the past two decades emphasizes the fact that we are part of nature; that we view it from the inside, and that we cannot study nature without studying ourselves as well.

As a matter of medical commonsense, there is a new and urgent emphasis on the setting in which we actually live our lives, on the conditions of life that we as a species have created for ourselves and on determining the limits of our ability to adapt to those conditions in reasonable ways.

As Hans Selye suggests, when you describe your own individual state as one of either sickness or health, you are describing the relationship between yourself and the world around you; the ability of your own system to adapt satisfactorily to the conditions under which you live your life, *and* the extent to which you have been able to take charge of those circumstances so as to maximize your adaptation.

Holism and the Health Sciences

It is often said that medicine itself is more an art than a science. There is something to the claim, even though we have been talking about medical science throughout this book. Any professional judgments about the best way to approach a particular medical problem must be made on the basis of the training and experience, and perhaps the talent, of the individual physician involved, and on the basis of the best information available to the physician at the time. But the solid information on which such judgments are based must come from the human sciences and the life sciences as well as from clinical and epidemiological research.

One reason it has been difficult to develop a comprehensive science of human health is that psychologists and endocrinologists, sociologists and pathologists, dieticians and microbiologists, simply do not come into close contact with each other. The scientific community is over-specialized and highly segmented, with no generally shared framework or vocabulary. It is even difficult for biologists to keep up with what other biologists are doing, let alone the interesting and possibly relevant things that psychologists might be doing. There are ten different biological fields recognized by the National

Academy of Sciences now, each with its own journals and professional associations, and thirteen other distinct sciences as well. Pulling together the many aspects of individual existence that are relevant to achieving and maintaining a healthy life will mean, first of all, opening channels of information among the scattered researchers. A general clearinghouse of information, perhaps under the aegis of the National Academy of Sciences, would be a good beginning. Research must be funded and encouraged to tie together the many areas of the human sciences into a comprehensive understanding of the influences on human health.

For psychology in particular, holism suggests a direction for new research. Our psychological characteristics are intimately connected to our biological history as a species, our individual experiences, and our physiological responses to daily events. The recent emphasis on the perceptual triggering of complex biochemical activity raises urgent questions of medical importance about the way we categorize our perceptions, both consciously and unconsciously, and about the individual contexts of expectation and experience in which we interpret our perceptions. Biology and psychology are concerned with many of the same events in human experience, but they describe those events from two different points of view, in much the same way that chemistry and physics often describe the same events from their distinct points of view. There is no reason to suppose that psychological theory can be replaced by biological description, any more than chemistry can be replaced by physics. But there is a need for a distinctly psychological understanding of those medically relevant aspects of human experience that determine how we adapt in both immediate and long-range ways to perceived changes in our surroundings, how efficiently we adapt, and how we can consciously set out to readjust our responses to events in our daily lives.

Behaviorism has been the dominant school of thought in American psychology for a long enough time that it has come to include both liberal and conservative factions. An over-simplified, cartoonish account of behaviorism holds that it treats the human organism as a black box whose innards are forever unknown. On the subject of perception, such a behaviorist can talk intelligibly about only the stimulus presented to a subject and the subject's response, with both described independently of the subject's (i.e. the black box's) understanding of them. The critics hold that the black box must be opened, that psychology must attend to the individual context of expectations, hopes and intentions that shapes the interpretation of stimuli and differentiates among the many possible reactions to them. Many of those reactions, as we have seen, are of direct relevance to health and resistance to disease. Understanding and eventually learning to modify the ways we react to changes in our environment will be a major goal of medical psychology over the next decade, and you can expect to see the arguments among psychologists heat up in this area.

In a similar vein, information about the arthritis-prone personality and the relationship between emotional history and cancer has been around for some time, but no one has known quite what to do with it. Attempts to use psychotherapy coupled with hypnosis and other altered states of consciousness to modify such emotional patterns are relatively new, as are the attempts to foster positive emotional attitudes as part of the treatment after surgery and in recuperation from serious illness. Jerome Frank's work on the role of "expectant faith" in healing virtually demonstrates that confidence is as much a physiological state as an emotional one. You can't describe both the conditions that inspire and foster such confidence and the effects of it on the person who feels it without using the whole vocabulary, including the vocabulary of emotions and intentions that the reductivist psychologists have never succeeded in replacing.

Respectability within the overall scientific community has not come easily to psychology, and a good part of the coming debate within the field is going to be about questions of method and evidence. When mechanism dominated physics and set the tone for proper scientific inquiry in the West, the study of overt "public" behavior was the one area open to psychologists where controlled experiment could be carried out at all. Any broadening of the methods of behavioristic psychology is still viewed with some suspicion within the discipline, where professionals are always on guard against the attitude that "anything goes" as a legitimate scientific method, as Berkeley philosopher Paul Feyerabend believes. Many conservative psychologists believe that the only alternatives to strict mechanism are mysticism and crackpottery.

But there are many areas of medicine where controlled experiment is simply not possible. Researchers must draw on the best available evidence from other sources: anecdotal reports of clinical experience, epidemiological studies of large populations, or even more indirect information. Controlled experiments are difficult or impossible to carry out in nutrition, or when the efficacy of specific medical or surgical treatments is being assessed. Evaluations of the reactions of individual patients to specific treatments is difficult to quantify—difficult to express in terms of measurable quantities so that one patient's rate of recovery can meaningfully be compared to another's. Preventive measures against disease are even harder to evaluate. Still, medical and surgical techniques can be, and are, critically evaluated on the basis of available anecdotal or statistical evidence, and determinations are made on the basis of informed professional judgment as to whether or not specific techniques are effective.

In this respect, holistic treatments like the Simontons' persuasive strategy against cancer are similar to surgical techniques; they can be evaluated only on the basis of clinical experience. They are in principle no more difficult to assess than other medical treatments. What has kept Western medicine from trying techniques like this in the past has not been a peculiar difficulty in evaluating them, but rather the fact that the strategies themselves seemed so implausible. The Simontons' work would have been dismissed as hocus pocus not too long ago, and it is still a matter of some controversy. Many professionals are skeptical, but many others are interested in it because it now has a ring of plausibility. The possible links between the strategy and the disease can now be sketched through the effects of emotional stimuli on neurochemistry and the presumed effect of neurochemical states on the triggering of the immune response and other natural complexes, such as the production of endorphins and steroids. Connections of this sort are still "not well understood," but the developing neurochemical research indicates what the explanations of such techniques are going to look like.

Dr. David S. Sobel, of the University of California's Health Policy Program, has called for the development of "a conceptual framework that bridges disciplinary, professional, and cultural boundaries."[159] There is every good reason to believe that such a synthesis is possible, and that it will take place as developments from distinct fields are brought together and discussed. And the recent respect for the techniques, if not for the theories, of the Eastern psychological disciplines promises to have a broadening effect on the theories of Western psychology. It isn't, as some suppose, that one approach to psychology is going to absorb or replace the other. The genuine successes of behaviorist psychology need to be integrated into a larger scheme of theory; there is no need to denigrate or discredit them. *What happens next* in Western psychology is likely to be influenced by both the success of behaviorism and the successes of the Eastern disciplines. A convergence of Eastern and Western scientific traditions in psychology is likely to take shape in what has been called a "cosmopolitan" approach to psychology and medicine.

What can we expect from the health sciences in the coming years? A gradual alteration of the existing structure of theory and practice to meet the critical challenge posed by new conceptions, new techniques, and new experimental results; not a wholesale and sudden abandonment of the sound methods that have become established in Western medicine. Following the direction pointed by Jerome Frank, Carl Simonton, Herbert Benson and others, you can expect to see an increased interest in the use of persuasive strategies to alter a person's attitudes toward disease and thereby improve the individual's ability to overcome disease and to recover from illness and injury. It is clear that events which are best described from an emotional, "mental" point of view can initiate a period of accelerated healing and recovery. The strategies used to manipulate those events will no doubt draw on the recent research into "altered states of consciousness," such as meditation and hypnosis. It is unrealistic to expect such holistic approaches to replace the use of medications or surgery. But they will no doubt culminate in the development of procedures that allow the treatment of specific disorders with *less* medication and *less* reliance on surgery.

We can also expect to hear a good deal more about the placebo effect. Many medical people have regarded the effectiveness of placebos as a sign that the ailments being treated were spurious to begin with. The conservative view on placebos has led to the conviction that it is absurd to try to *manipulate* the placebo effect as part of the medical treatment for illness. But the work of Jerome Frank on faith healing, and the more recent studies carried out on the placebo effect by Herbert Benson at Harvard and Jon Levine in California, indicate that *belief* in the placebo may work in very specific ways to stimulate the natural spontaneous production of endorphins to deal with pain, and steroids to deal with inflammation. Medical scientists are eager to learn more about the physiology of the placebo effect, about the way in which thought processes can alter physiology in definable and reproducible ways. Benson, whose work on the relaxation response has already had considerable impact, has recently begun a research project to study the healing practices of other eras and cultures, with the hope of ferreting out further techniques for manipulating the human system's own capacities for healing. It is reasonable to expect development of further persuasive strategies that can be used as adjuncts to medication and surgery in the treatment of heart disease, high blood pressure, and cancer.

At the same time, research along more traditional lines will continue. The multifaceted attack on the problem of cancer will involve further research at the cellular level to determine the local nature of the disease, and at the systemic level to determine the extent to which both physiological and persuasive stimulation of the immune response can be used as a means of intervention in the course of the disease.

Lewis Thomas believes that a single, straightforward cause-and-cure eventually will be found for cancer. Many other researchers believe that there is no such single line of approach to be found. I suspect that this disagreement is a matter of emphasis; that at a level of abstraction far removed from the events of ordinary life, a single set of cellular characteristics associated with cancer can be discussed. But there are no medical or surgical treatments at the cellular level, and no ways to manipulate cellular events in such a way as to safeguard against cancer. At the level of everyday events that you and I can do something about, there are indefinitely many sets of circumstances that can affect the rate at which we generate abnormal cells, and just as many that can affect our ability to weed out and destroy such cells by means of our immune systems. Further work in epidemiology and the detection of carcinogenic substances *and habits* is to be expected.

The holistic emphasis on our biological heritage, and on our ancestors' relationship to their environment as compared with our relationship to our own environment, will open up new lines of argument concerning human nature and human needs. A case in point is the line of reasoning used by Pauling and Stone, estimating our optimum intake of ascorbic acid on the basis of the available information about our ancestors' eating habits, and on the basis of ascorbic acid production in other species. Since nutritional needs are so hard to measure, it becomes legitimate to look for such indirect evidence about the nature of those needs. It becomes reasonable to ask some distinctly anthropological questions about how our nutritional needs developed, and to draw inferences about our adaptive responses by considering the ways in which our ancestors had to adapt to the conditions of primitive life. In psychology, there has recently been a revival of a movement called "organicism" that is distinctly holistic, and that attempts to approach psychological questions by means of a study of our adaptive capacities and the biological history of the species.

As recently as the mid-seventies, coming out in favor of holism in medical research and care was like joining the underground. Now holism is well represented within the mainstream of medical research. I sincerely believe that holistic questions are going to dominate medical and psychological research over the next few years. The anti-scientific extremists on the one side, and the mechanistic conservatives on the other, are becoming fewer and fewer. More people in the medical professions have come to respect both approaches to the prevention and treatment of the major diseases of civilization. The impact of holism on the health sciences has been to broaden the scope of mainstream research, not to exclude any well-established approaches to disease.

Holism and Medical Care

The change in thinking that holism represents doesn't mean that you have to find yourself a new doctor, or that you should start avoiding the medical profession altogether. A reasonable approach to the new insights of holism must include a sense of continuity with the long and successful tradition of scientific medicine. The problem for any medical practitioner is to decide just how drastically to intervene in a person's own battle against disease, which of the available techniques to use, and where to intervene in the complicated chain of events that constitute the human system's own means for self-defense. On the one hand there is a long-established expectation that if a person is "really sick" then what is called for is intervention, at least in the form of prescription medicine. We, the consumers of medical services, have come to expect medication and surgery as the only acceptable ways to deal with genuine illness. This belief is reflected in the benefit schedules of most medical insurance programs, and it influences the kind of treatment that many doctors offer their patients. On the other hand, there is growing protest against the unnecessary reliance on medical and surgical intervention.

This much is clear now: holistic techniques which involve changes in personal habits, psychological approaches, and the use of persuasive strategies, can lessen our reliance on medication and surgery. Whether or not the sole treatment for a specific ailment can be holistic in this sense is another matter. You can expect that research on such questions will be reported widely in the coming years, and it is reasonable to expect your family physician to be informed about such research. But in every case, an informed professional is obligated to choose the best mode of treatment that is available at the time, and that has been demonstrated to be safe and reliable. The best available treatment for your ailment at the time you have it might turn out to be the traditional one.

Don't just throw away your pills if you are already taking prescribed medication. There is a good possibility that you will be able to reduce or eliminate medication for some conditions if you change your personal habits or learn a technique for self-regulation. But you have to develop the new habits first, and be sure that you can maintain them. Don't expect to eliminate medical problems by simply willing them away. It isn't that easy. It requires determination and effort to control high blood pressure and other medical problems by the alteration of personal habit. Deciding to take charge of a problem is something different from pretending that the problem doesn't exist. You should expect your doctor to caution you about the many fads that will arise in the name of holism. But if you make it clear that you are looking for solutions to your medical problems in a serious and sensible way, you can generally enlist your doctor's help in your efforts at self-regulation.

Your physician is as much an individual as you are. Differences in training and experience which have nothing to do with competence lead to reasonable differences among physicians in the way they treat specific illnesses, as well as the way they conduct diagnostic examinations and how much advice they give about matters of diet, exercise, and personal habit. There are "movement" doctors who are very much concerned about self-care and stress relief, about advising patients on diet and exercise. And there are doctors who are no less competent who prefer to reserve all advice unless there is a clearly definable ailment that can be treated by medication in the traditional manner. Most family physicians probably fall somewhere in between. This reflects legitimate differences in medical philosophy among professionals, in the overall view of what counts as a sound and responsible practice of medicine. It is reasonable to seek out a family physician whose philosophy of medicine is like your own, to ask any physician about alternatives to medication and surgery, and to accept informed professional judgment about your treatment.

Journalist Norman Cousins has had dramatic personal experience with a disease that responded ultimately to massive pharmacological doses of ascorbic acid and a persuasive technique that entailed inducing laughter.[39] Based on his own experience, Cousins suggests what it is reasonable to expect of your family physician.[40] You should expect, for example, that your physician will keep an open mind about new developments in diagnosis and treatment, and keep informed about clinical research into new techniques such as biofeedback, meditation, autogenic training, and altering diet and personal habits in order to deal with specific disorders, rather than resorting immediately to medication. But you should not expect your physician to use or recommend any treatment you may have heard about unless he is convinced that there is clear clinical evidence of its safety and effectiveness.

If you let your physician know that you would prefer to approach medical matters by adjusting your personal habits wherever that is possible, he should be willing to cooperate. If your physician feels that such an approach is inappropriate in your case, it is reasonable to expect him to tell you why.

Suppose, for example, that at the time of your regular checkup, one of the physiological measurements is slightly outside normal limits: uric acid is slightly elevated, say, indicating perhaps the early stages of gout; or serum cholesterol is slightly above normal limits; or your blood pressure is a bit higher than it usually is—say 135/92. With such minor deviations, it is reasonable to expect your physician to discuss adjustments in your eating habits or your ways of dealing with stress that might change the situation, to give you a list of foods to cut back on or to avoid altogether *before* resorting to medication or, alternatively, to explain why medication is preferable immediately in your particular case.

In the instance of a slight elevation in blood pressure, it is reasonable to expect your physician to discuss your suggestion that you try the relaxation response as a means of dealing with it. He may propose a deal, as my physician recently did: try it for a few weeks and then let's check the blood pressure again. If it hasn't improved, he may insist on medication. That is a fair and prudent deal. If your doctor won't agree to it, he should tell you why *in your case* it would be inappropriate, or why he doubts the widely accepted results of studies such as those by Herbert Benson and the group at Harvard University Medical School. But if your doctor ridicules the idea or dismisses it out of hand, you might want to seek another opinion.

As Cousins suggests, it is reasonable to expect your physician to be concerned about your nutritional habits and to ask about them as an essential part of any examination. And it is reasonable to expect him to accept the need for vitamin supplementation, especially if you are under stress or if the circumstances of your life subject you to environmental strains or hazards. But it isn't at all reasonable to expect your physician to accept the simplistic notion that all diseases are the manifestations of vitamin deficiencies, or that the right foods will cure every known disease. Expect him to caution you about the dangers of vitamin overdose and about the waste involved in taking excessive amounts of vitamins. Seek your doctor's advice about your individual attempts to steer a sensible course between the extremes.

Finally, you should expect your physician to deal with you as a person, not as an isolated set of symptoms, and to consider your illness as an occurrence in your individual life. You can expect him to discuss with you matters of personal habit and hygiene that may have led to the illness, and the alterations of personal habit that may help you to recover from it. Physicians as well as patients have to assume a new kind of responsibility in dealing with illness.

Holism and Your Lifestyle

There is no finite list of things that you can and must do to improve your adjustment to the circumstances of your life, or to assure that you will maintain a state of good health. There is rather a constant round of small decisions about day-to-day living, and these decisions will, as always, be governed by your views of yourself and the world. Most of us can't escape the pressures and other health hazards of modern life. What we have to do instead is find effective ways to deal with them. This means coming to an understanding of our own nature as persons—not as mechanisms to be adjusted, oiled, fueled, and occasionally repaired, but as organisms with capabilities and limitations rooted in our biological history. We need to be aware that our systems respond to events as we interpret them, and that we ourselves generate many of the signals that initiate involuntary activities which can affect our health in both positive and negative ways.

We learn how to interpret events around us, how to live and how to take care of ourselves, how to pace ourselves and how to nourish ourselves. To change an unsatisfactory adjustment to the facts of our individual lives requires some relearning, not a patchwork of emergency measures designed to deal with the results of a bad adjustment.

The difficulty comes when you ask where to turn for guidance. Health fads have been around for as long as people have been concerned about health. At times like the present, when medical thinking is changing rapidly, the health fads increase. It is difficult for an individual to sort out the sound from the unsound, to differentiate the approach to diet that just might have something to it from the dangerous food fads that can actually kill people. The frustrating fact that precise dietary requirements cannot be nailed down leads many people to listen to those who claim on the basis of little or no evidence that they have found the unique way to guarantee proper nutrition and good health. Beware of such claims for uniqueness, and beware of simplistic approaches that claim to be right for everyone.

In general, it is foolish to alter your eating habits, or any other habits, on the basis of claims that are not backed by formal research. And even then, a press release about a single clinical study should not be taken as an argument for a drastic change in your way of living. It took a number of clinical studies to establish the hazards of saccharine, and fully ten years to establish a convincing argument in favor of dietary supplementation with ascorbic acid.

Unless your physician specifically recommends a restricted diet as a means for dealing with an ailment, it is clearly best to reject any dietary plan which excludes whole groups of foods. The nutrition research discussed earlier shows clearly that the greater the variety in your diet, the better off you are. In general, the epidemiological studies which link some eating habits with an increased risk of cancer constitute arguments for reducing or adjusting the amounts of the foods in question in your diet, not for eliminating them altogether. Such studies reveal the consequences of dietary habits which concentrate too heavily on one kind of food.

Beware also of the "alien culture" fads which try to duplicate the lifestyles of other cultures and times. Suggestions that you should base your food choices on the habits of fifteenth-century sheepherders in the Asiatic highlands are generally foolish and expensive. The differences in daily activity and in the kinds of food available to us make such arguments irrelevant to contemporary life. A "cosmopolitan" approach is better: by all means *broaden* your choices by incorporating unfamiliar foods as they come on the market—bean sprouts and the many nourishing products of soybeans that are staples of Oriental diets can increase the variety in your own menus—but don't restrict your choices to these things.

And beware of claims that there is one special food that will guarantee you good health. The yogurt advertisements which suggest that we can live as long as a group of middle-European village people if we eat as much yogurt as they do should be taken with good humor. Yogurt is a wholesome and nourishing food, but its presence in the diet of these long-lived people is only one element in a total lifestyle. We can learn something by studying the habits of such groups of people, but we probably cannot accomplish much by trying to duplicate their diets. Their longevity is no doubt due to a very local combination of conditions which include the climate, the minerals in the water supply, their habits of activity and, not least of all, genetic factors, in addition to their diet.

Your best guidance still comes from the professionals, from summations of epidemiological evidence rather than from single statistical comparisons, from arguments based on clinical testing where that is available, and from arguments that draw upon what is known of our biological heritage. You can expect to hear a good deal about our primitive ancestors and what we know of their habits, because our own biological needs are rooted in theirs. Examinations of the teeth of prehistoric skeletons to determine whether or not our early ancestors ate meat (they did) have some bearing on the question whether or not our diets should include animal proteins.

Most of us do not produce our own foodstuffs, and we have no direct access to the people who do. We must rely on public policy and government agencies to insure the safety of the food supply, and the regulations are not always as clear or as strict as we would like. The bureaucracy often responds to pressures other than those which have to do with the health of the public. It is still possible for additives to be introduced into processed foods without exhaustive testing to determine the effects of those additives on the human system, although there has recently been effective pressure from the medical professions and the public for a tightening of the regulations. The priorities which determine the actions of food processors are different from the priorities of the consumer. Foods that keep well and are easily shipped are not always the most nourishing. Additives that make possible the economical processing of foods may diminish the nutritive value of those foods, or may even constitute a direct danger to health. There are two things to be done about this: one political, and the other economic. On the political side, the more of us who lend our voices to the demand for testing and regulation of food additives, the better off we will be. On the economic side, you can contribute to the pressure for safe food processing by being careful about what you buy. Whatever the government regulations are at a given time, the burden of proof must rest with the manufacturer who claims that a given food additive can safely be introduced into the food supply. It isn't up to us to show that a given additive is dangerous; it is up to the producers and the regulatory agencies to provide us with good reason to believe that it is safe. In the interest of both economy and safety, it is generally best to concentrate on fresh, unprocessed foods. If you use precooked or processed foods, read the labels. A surprising number of canned and frozen foods on the market contain no additives at all. If there is anything on the list of ingredients that you don't recognize or don't have good reason to believe to be safe, don't buy the product. Such a practice demands that you learn something about food preservation and the functions of such organic additives as lecithin, which is a product of soybeans and a legitimate emulsifying additive to keep sauces and mixtures intact in transit.

Labeling laws have improved in the past few years; there is a continuing effort to raise the standards of testing and to test those products used in food preparation, like the nitrites used in smoked meats, which came into common use before the current concern about such matters. Constant public pressure on regulatory agencies to impose strict testing standards on all elements of food production and processing is going to have results.

The problem of a polluted environment is not going to go away quickly, if it goes away at all. The dangers to health imposed by the needs of industry are complicated by political and economic considerations. There have been, and will continue to be, trade-offs between the public needs which are met by specific industrial practices and the consequences of those practices on the air, water, and food supplies, as well as the levels of ambient radiation in our surroundings. The political realities of industrial pollution may well condemn us all, as some people believe. Again, the best line of attack on such problems is political: pressure for zoning regulations, pressure for the testing of industrial byproducts to assure their safety and regulation of the amounts of pollutants that can be released. Such matters will increasingly become issues of public policy that will figure in local and national elections. What we, as individuals, can do is stay informed and become increasingly vocal.

Somewhere between the extremes of the back-to-nature faddists who insist that all the trappings of modern life must be done away with, and the plastic culture faddists who are willing to ignore health hazards in the interests of convenience and profit, there is a sane course to steer, and all of us are looking for it. We are aware of the need to re-adjust our thinking and our expectations. The principle identified as "Appropriate Technology" has begun to take hold in public life, as the Congress pays more attention to expenditures for equipment and technical resources requested by governmental agencies. It has becme a consideration in private life, too, as many of us have had to think about the ways in which we use energy in our homes and in transportation. This is a time of transition from a heedless increase in unnecessary gadgetry to a more sensible approach to a level of technology that meets human needs and at the same time is frugal with scarce resources, unintrusive on the environment, and manageable with reasonable economy. The fact that such matters are being addressed publicly and responsibly indicates a new awareness of the relevance of a balanced technology to our well-being. Taking charge of your own health means making your voice heard politically and economically, as well as regulating your personal habits. The health policies that you support with your vote, the products that you buy, and the products you refuse to buy, can have an impact.

Apart from making sensible decisions about foods and environmental matters, your individual habits and responsibilities are the most important part of a holistic scheme of living. It seems better in this area to emphasize what you are seeking rather than what you are avoiding. Life should not be a long series of prohibitions. Things aren't that bad yet, and they may never be. We need to stay away from the extremes of a morbid preoccupation with disease and bodily functions on the one hand, and a total disregard for the biological limits of human tolerance on the other. Sensible habits of nutrition, rest, exercise, stress relief, medical checkups and preventive health measures need not be particularly severe or filled with prohibitions, or even with rigid imperatives. And again, there is no package deal that is going to be appropriate for everyone; you have to make individual decisions about the needs of your own lifestyle.

Take exercise, for example. Most of us know that we have a biological need for physical activity, but it is all too easy to fall into sedentary habits. Moreover, some people just can't sustain an interest in doing exercises for their own sake. The thought of sit-ups, jogging, or even minor sports, is repellent to them. If you are such a person, then it would be sensible to try to include more physical exertion in the things that you would be doing in any case. A five-minute errand in the car might become a twenty-minute errand that involves a brisk walk— the kind where, as one doctor puts it, "you stand up straight, suck in your gut, and stretch your legs." A little creative thinking can turn up a number of minor chores in your daily routine that can be done as well by muscle power as by motor power, with benefits in both overall economy and exercise.

Now that behavioral means for dealing with stress have been subjected to clinical study with positive results, it is worthwhile to learn at least one of the available techniques so that you can let down without needing to resort to drugs or alcohol. The way that works for you may or may not be some form of meditation, but the basic technique in one of the many variants mentioned earlier is worth a try. There is no longer any reasonable ground to doubt that eliciting the relaxation response on a regular basis can be beneficial to both your health and your outlook.

Taking charge of your own welfare means learning how to manage stress before something serious, like hypertension, develops. We cannot live irresponsibly and expect to depend upon medical miracles to bail us out when we get ourselves in trouble. There are no such medical miracles. None of the ways for repairing organic damage through surgery, medication, or other therapy can guarantee that you will be able to avoid serious illness for the rest of your life, and it is clear that even the most sophisticated and informed holistic program can make no such guarantee either. What the holistic emphasis does provide is an expanded basis for improving our ability to cope effectively with the needs of contemporary living so as to increase the likelihood of a long and healthy life, to minimize the risk of serious disease, and to enable us to deal with disease more effectively when it does occur.

In some cases, it will be necessary to seek professional help in changing habits of tension and stress. That doesn't mean that you can expect professionals to solve every problem for you, but rather that you can legitimately expect them to show you how to take charge of your own states. Biofeedback, meditation, and other techniques are easily available to most of us.

Regular physical checkups are best thought of as a kind of biofeedback. They entail monitoring such physiological states as the composition of the blood and the state of internal organs—things of which we aren't generally aware through direct sensory signals. The question to be asked in your physical is "How am I doing?" rather that "What's wrong with me?" And the aim is to find areas where we need to fine-tune our adjustment to the circumstances we live in.

Probably most important of all is the attitude of *taking charge* in informed, responsible ways. Most of us are not the helpless victims of circumstances; we are responsible for what we settle for in life, for the compromises we make and the habits we develop. It does matter how you think and what you believe. It matters how you feel about yourself and how you take charge of your circumstances. The psychological studies of people who contract arthritis, cancer, and heart disease, coupled with the new understanding of the biology of human emotion, show just how much those things matter. The relevance of our attitudes, reactions, and emotional habits to the state of our health is perhaps the most important single insight to come out of the conceptual change from dualism to holism.

It matters how you think of yourself. It is no longer reasonable to think of your body as a thing that you either do or don't take care of. There is no clear distinction to be drawn between you and your body. You are a person, a biological unit, and every habit you have is a measure of how well you are suited to live in the world around you. If you begin with the assumption that you are *supposed* to be healthy all the time, and you understand this in terms of your own responsibility for coping effectively with the conditions of your individual life, then you have already increased the likelihood that you can remain healthy. In most cases, health and illness are not matters of chance, not things that happen to us because of forces outside our control, but conditions that we create for ourselves. The will to live, the will to be healthy, the willingness to take charge of our own lives and our habits, and the acceptance of the responsibility for making informed decisions about the circumstances in which we live our lives, all come together in a holistic picture of sensible living. In the final analysis, we ourselves determine the course of our lives. Good health is a state of a whole person.

REFERENCES

1. Achterberg, J.; Matthews-Simonton, S.; and Simonton, O. C. "Psychology of the Exceptional Cancer Patient: A Description of Patients Who Outlive Predicted Life-Expectancies." *Psychotherapy: Theory, Research and Practice,* 1977, *14,* 416–22.

2. Agren, Hans. "Patterns of Tradition and Modernization in Contemporary Chinese Medicine. In *Medicine in Chinese Cultures,* ed. Arthur Kleinman et al., pp. 37–59. USDHEW, 1975.

3. Ames, Bruce N. Identifying Environmental Chemicals Causing Mutations and Cancer. *Science,* 11 May 1979, 587–93.

4. Amkraut, A., and Solomon, G. F. "From the Symbolic Stimulus to the Pathophysiologic Response: Immune Mechanisms." *International Journal of Psychiatry in Medicine,* 1975, 5, 541–63.

5. Anand, B. W.; Chhina, G. S.; and Singh, B. "Some Aspects of Electroencephalographic Studies in Yogis." *Electroencephalography and Clinical Neurophysiology,* 1961, *13,* 452–56. Reprinted in *Altered States of Consciousness,* C. T. Tart, ed. New York: John Wiley and Sons, 1969, pp. 503–6.

6. Anderson, E. E., and Anderson M. L. "Folk Dietetics in Two Chinese Communities, and Its Implications for the Study of Chinese Medicine." In *Medicine in Chinese Cultures,* ed. Arthur Kleinman et al., pp. 143–75. USDHEW, 1975.

7. Anderson, Terrence W. et al. "Vitamin C and the Common Cold: A Double-Blind Trial." *Canadian Medical Association Journal,* 1972, *107,* 503–08.

8. Ardrey, Robert. *The Social Contract.* New York: Atheneum, 1970.

9. Bahnson, C. B. "Psychophysiological Complementarity in Malignancies: Past Work and Future Vistas." *Annals of the New York Academy of Sciences,* 1969, *164,* 319–34.

10. ———. "Basic Epistemological Considerations Regarding Psychosomatic Processes and Their Application to Current Psychophysiological Cancer Research." *International Journal of Psychobiology,* 1970, *1,* 57–69.

11. ———and Bahnson, M. B. "The Role of Ego Defenses: Denial and Repression in the Etiology of Malignant Neoplasm." *Annals of the New York Academy of Sciences,* 1966, *125,* 827–45.

12. ———. "Ego Defenses in Cancer Patients." *Annals of the New York Academy of Sciences,* 1969, *164,* 546–49.

13. Barber, T. X.; DiCara, L. V.; Kamita, J.; Miller, N. E.; Shapiro, D.; and Stoyva, J., eds. *Biofeedback and Self-Control 1970.* Chicago: Aldine-Atherton, 1971.

14. Barchas, J. D.; Akil, H.; Elliott, G. R.; Holman, R. B.; and Watson, S. J. "Behavioral Neurochemistry: Neuroregulators and Behavioral States." *Science,* 1978, *200,* 964–73.

15. Beach, Nancy. "Variety: The Spice of a Well-balanced Diet." *New York Times Magazine,* January 28, 1979, 60–63.

16. Beisel, W. R. "Malnutrition as a Consequence of Stress." In *Malnutrition and the Immune Response,* R. M. Suskind, ed. New York: Raven, 1977.

17. Benson, Herbert (with Miriam Z. Klipper). *The Relaxation Response.* New York: William Morrow, 1975.

18. Berger, Philip A. "Medical Treatment of Mental Illness." *Science,* 1978, *200,* 974–81.

19. Berkley, George E. *Cancer.* Englewood Cliffs, N.J.: Prentice-Hall, 1978.

20. Blumberg, E. T.; West, R. M.; and Ellis, F. W. "A Possible Relationship Between Psychological Factors and Cancer." *Psychosomatic Medicine,* 1954, *16,* 194–98.

21. Boyd, W. *The Spontaneous Regression of Cancer.* Springfield, Ill.: Charles C. Thomas, 1966.

22. Breslow, L. "Risk Factor Intervention for Health Maintenance." *Science,* 1978, *200,* 908–12.

23. Brown, Barbara B. *Stress and the Art of Biofeedback.* New York: Harper and Row, 1977.

24. Bruner, Jerome. "On Perceptual Readiness." *Psychological Review,* 1957, *64,* 123–52.

25. Bunker, J. P.; Barnes, B. A.; Mosteller, F., eds. *Costs, Risks and Benefits of Surgery.* New York: Oxford University Press, 1977.

26. Bunker, J. P.; Hinkley, D.; and McDermott, W. V. "Surgical Innovation and Its Evaluation." *Science,* 1978, *200,* 937–41.

27. Burkitt, Denis P. "The Link Between Low-Fiber Diets and Disease." *Human Nature,* December 1978, 34–41.

28. Burnet, F. M. *Immunological Surveillance.* New York: Pergamon Press, 1970.

29. ———, ed. *Immunology*. San Francisco: Freeman, 1976.

30. Burrows, William. "The Cancer Safety Controversy." *The New York Times Magazine*, March 25, 1979, 82–85.

31. Cameron, E.; and Pauling, L. "Ascorbic Acid and the Glycosaminoglycans: An Orthomolecular Approach to Cancer and Other Diseases." *Oncology*, 1973, *27*, 181.

32. ———. "The Orthomolecular Treatment of Cancer: I. The Role of Ascorbic Acid in Host Resistance." *Chemical Biological Interaction*, 1974, *9*, 273.

33. Carlson, Rick J. "The End of Medicine." In *Conference on Future Directions in Health Care: The Dimensions of Medicine*. Knowles, J. H.; Lee, P. R.; and McNerney, W. J., eds. New York, 1975. Sponsored by The Rockefeller Foundation, Blue Cross Assn., and the Health Policy Program, The University of California at San Francisco.

34. Chandra, R. K.; and Newberne, P. M. *Nutrition, Immunity, and Infection: Mechanisms and Interactions*. New York: Plenum Press, 1977.

35. "The Chemistry of Acupuncture." *Scientific American*, July 1979, 79–80.

36. Chen, Ronald. *The History and Methods of Physical Diagnosis in Classical Chinese Medicine*. New York: Vantage Press, 1969.

37. Cheraskin, E., and Ringsdorf, W. M., Jr. (with Arlene Brecher). *Psychodietetics: Food as the Key to Emotional Health*. Briarcliff Manor, N.Y.: Stein and Day, 1974, Reprint, New York: Bantam Books, 1976.

38. Comroe, Julius H. Jr. "The Road from Research to New Diagnosis and Therapy." *Science*, 1978, *200*, 931–37.

39. Cousins, Norman. *Anatomy of an Illness as Perceived by the Patient*. New York: W. W. Norton, 1979.

40. ———. "The Holistic Health Explosion." *Saturday Review*, March 31, 1979, 17–20.

41. Croce, Carlo M.; and Koprowski, Hilary. "The Genetics of Human Cancer." *Scientific American*, February 1978, 117–25.

42. Crombie, A. C. "Early Concepts of the Senses and the Mind." *Scientific American*, May 1964, 108–16.

43. Currie, G. A. "Eighty Years of Immunotherapy: A Review of Immunological Methods Used for the Treatment of Human Cancer." *British Journal of Cancer*, 1972, *26*, 141.

44. Devoret, Raymond. "Bacterial Tests for Potential Carcinogens." *Scientific American*, August 1979, 40–49.

45. DiCara, L. V., and Miller, N. E. "Instrumental Learning of Systolic Blood Pressure Responses by Curarized Rats: Dissociation of Cardiac and Vascular Changes." *Psychosomatic Medicine,* 1968, *30,* 489–94.

46. ———. "Heart-rate Learning in the Noncurarized State, Transfer to the Curarized State, and Subsequent Retraining in the Noncurarized State." *Psychology of Behavior,* 1969, *4,* 621–24.

47. Dobzhansky, Theodosius. *Mankind Evolving: The Evolution of the Human Species.* New Haven: Yale University Press, 1962.

48. Dubos, Rene. "Health and Creative Adaptation." *Human Nature,* January 1978, 74–82.

49. ———. "Medicine Evolving." In *Ways of Health,* ed. D. S. Sobel. New York: Harcourt Brace Jovanovich, 1979.

50. Duke, Marc. *Acupuncture.* New York: Pyramid Books, 1973.

51. Dunn, Fred L. "Traditional Asian Medicine and Cosmopolitan Medicine as Adaptive Systems." In *Asian Medical Systems,* ed. C. Leslie. Berkeley: University of California Press, 1976.

52. Everson, T. C., and Cole, W. H. *Spontaneous Regression of Cancer.* Philadelphia: W. B. Saunders, 1966.

53. Farquhar, J. W. et al. *Lancet,* 1977, *1,* 1192.

54. Fehmi, Lester. "Open Focus Training." Paper delivered at the annual meeting of the Biofeedback Research Society, February 5, 1975.

55. Feigl, Herbert. *The "Mental" and the "Physical": The Essay and a Postscript.* Minneapolis: University of Minnesota Press, 1967.

56. Fiore, Neil, Ph.D. "Fighting Cancer: One Patient's Perspective." *The New England Journal of Medicine,* February 8, 1979, *300,* 284–89.

57. Frank, Jerome D. *Persuasion and Healing: A Comparative Study of Psychotherapy.* New York: Schocken Books, 1963; rev. ed. 1974.

58. ———. "The Faith that Heals." *The Johns Hopkins Medical Journal,* 1975, *137,* 127–31.

59. ———. "Holistic Approaches to Health Care: The Concept." In *Conference on Future Directions in Health Care: The Dimensions of Medicine.* Knowles, J. H.; Lee, P. R.; and McNerney, W. J., eds. New York, 1975.

60. ———. "Nonmedical Healing: Religious and Secular." In *Ways of Health,* D. S. Sobel, ed. New York: Harcourt Brace Jovanovich, 1979.

61. Frankel, Fred H. *Hypnosis: Trance as a Coping Mechanism.* New York: Plenum Medical Book Co., 1976.

62. Frazier, Howard S., and Hiatt, Howard H. "Evaluation of Medical Practices." *Science,* 1978, *200,* 875–78.

63. Gengerelli, J. A., and Kirkner, F. J., eds. *Psychological Variables in Human Cancer.* Berkeley and Los Angeles: University of California Press, 1954.

64. Gillie, Oliver. "New Clues to Cancer." *Atlas World Press Review,* January 1977. Reprinted from the *Sunday Times,* London, June 13, 1976.

65. Glasser, Ronald J. *The Body is the Hero.* New York: Random House, 1976.

66. Gleidman, L. H.; Nash, E. H., Jr.; Imber, S. D.; Stone, A. R.; and Frank, J. D. "Reduction of Symptoms by Pharmacologically Inert Substances and by Short-term Psychotherapy." *Archives of Neurology and Psychiatry,* 1958, *79,* 345–51.

67. Grad, Bernard. "Healing by the Laying on of Hands: A Review of Experiments." In *Ways of Health,* D. S. Sobel, ed. New York: Harcourt Brace Jovanovich, 1979.

68. Gray, Jeffrey A. "Anxiety." *Human Nature,* July 1978, 38–45.

69. Green, Elmer, and Green, Alyce. *Beyond Biofeedback.* New York: Dell, 1977.

70. Haggard, Howard W. *Devils, Drugs and Doctors.* New York: Harper and Bros., 1929.

71. Hamburg, David A., and Brown, Sarah S. "The Science Base and Social Context of Health Maintenance: An Overview." *Science,* 1978, *200,* 847–49.

72. Hartmann, Ernst. "Tryptophane." *Archives of General Psychiatry,* September 1974.

73. Hess, Walter R. *The Functional Organization of the Diencephalon.* New York: Greene and Stratton, 1957.

74. Hilgard, Ernest R., and Hilgard, Josephine R. *Hypnosis in the Relief of Pain.* Los Altos, Calif.: William Kaufmann, 1975.

75. Hixson, J. R. "Interferon: It Interferes with Disease." *Science Digest,* September 1978, 18–22.

76. Holmes, T. H., and Rahe, R. H. "The Social Readjustment Rating Scale." *Journal of Psychosomatic Research,* 1967, *11,* 213.

77. Holzer, Hans. *Beyond Medicine.* Chicago: Henry Regnery Co., 1973.

78. Hutschnecker, Arnold A. *The Will to Live.* New York: Crowell, 1953.

79. "Jogging for the Mind." *Time,* July 24, 1978, 42.
80. Johnston, R. B., and Stroud, R. M. "Complement and Host Defense Against Infection." *Journal of Pediatrics,* 1977, *90,* 169.
81. Josephy, H. "Analysis of Mortality and Causes of Death in a Mental Hospital." *American Journal of Psychiatry,* 1949, *106,* 185–89.
82. Karlowski, T. R. et al. "Ascorbic Acid for the Common Cold: A Prophylactic and Therapeutic Trial." *Journal of the American Medical Association,* March 10, 1975, *231,* 1038–42.
83. Kasamatsu, Akira, and Hirai, Tomio. "An Electroencephalographic Study on the Zen Meditation (Zazen)." *Folio Psychiat. and Neurolog. Japonica,* 1966, *20,* 315–36. Reprinted in *Altered States of Consciousness,* ed. C. T. Tart. New York: John Wiley and Sons, 1969.
84. Kaslof, Leslie J., ed. *Wholistic Dimensions of Healing: A Resource Guide.* New York: Doubleday, 1979.
85. ———. "Holistic Medicine" (letter to the editor). *The New England Journal of Medicine,* May 24, 1979, *300,* 1221.
86. Kennedy, Donald. "What Animal Research Says About Cancer." *Human Nature,* May 1978, 84–89.
87. Kleinman, Arthur; Kunstadter, Peter; Alexander, E. R.; and Gale, James L., eds. *Medicine in Chinese Cultures: Comparative Studies of Health Care in Chinese and Other Societies.* U.S. Department of Health, Education, and Welfare: DHEW Publication Number (NIH) 75–653, 1975.
88. Kleinman, Arthur. "The Failure of Western Medicine." *Human Nature,* November 1978, 63–68.
89. Koestler, Arthur. *The Act of Creation.* New York: Macmillan, 1969.
90. Kolata, Gina Bari. Mental Disorders: A New Approach to Treatment?" *Science,* 1979, *203,* 36–38.
91. Körner, Stephan. *Experience and Theory.* London: Routledge and Kegan Paul, 1966.
92. Krahenbuhl, James L., and Remington, Jack S. "Belligerent Blood Cells: Immunotherapy and Cancer." *Human Nature,* January 1978, 52–59.
93. Krieg, Margaret B. *Green Medicine: The Search for Plants that Heal.* Chicago: Rand McNally, 1964.
94. Kroger, W. S. "Hypnotism and Acupuncture." *Journal of the American Medical Association,* 1972, *220,* 1012–13.
95. Lambo, T. A. "Psychotherapy in Africa." *Human Nature,* March 1978, 32–39.

96. LeShan, L. "An Emotional Life-History Pattern Associated with Neoplastic Disease." *Annals of the New York Academy of Sciences,* 1960, *125,* 780–93.

97. ———, and Worthington, R. E. "Some Recurrent Life History Patterns Observed in Patients with Malignant Disease. *Journal of Nervous and Mental Disorders,* 1956, *124,* 460–65.

98. Leslie, Charles, ed. *Asian Medical Systems: A Comparative Study.* Berkeley: University of California Press, 1976.

99. Levi, L. ed. *Emotions: Their Parameters and Measurement.* New York: Raven Press, 1975.

100. ———. *Society, Stress and Disease: The Psychosocial Environment and Psychosomatic Disease,* vol. I. London: Oxford University Press, 1974.

101. Luthe, Wolfgang. "Autogenic Training: Method, Research and Application in Medicine." *American Journal of Psychotherapy,* 1963, *17,* 174–95. Reprinted in *Altered States of Consciousness,* ed. Charles T. Tart. New York: John Wiley and Sons, 1969.

102. Maccoby, N.; Farquhar, Wood, P. D.; and Alexander, J. *Journal of Community Health,* Winter 1977, *3,* 100.

103. MacSweeney, David A. "Treatment of Unipolar Depression." *Lancet,* 13 September 1975, *2,* 510.

104. Man, P. le, and Chen, C. H. "Acupuncture anesthesia: A New Theory and Clinical Study." *Current Therapeutic Research,* 1972, *14,* 390–94.

105. Manaka, Yoshio, and Urquhart, I. A. *The Layman's Guide to Acupuncture.* New York: Weatherhill, 1972.

106. Margolis, Joseph. *Persons and Minds: The Prospects of Nonreductive Materialism.* Dordrecht and Boston: D. Reidel, 1978.

107. Marocco, N., and Rigotti, E. "Kidney Protective Effect of Vitamin C in Arsenic Poisoning." *Minerva Urologica,* 1962, *14,* 207–12.

108. Marx, Jean L. "Antibodies (I): New Information About Gene Structure." *Science,* 1978, *202,* 298–99.

109. ———. "Interferon (I): On the Threshold of Clinical Application." *Science,* 15 June 1979, 1183–86.

110. McKeown, Pat. "Does the Body Hold a Cancer Cure?" *Philadelphia Bulletin,* January 14, 1969, 1, 8.

111. McKeown, Thomas. *The Modern Rise of Population.* New York: Academic Press, 1976.

112. ———. 1978. "Determinants of Health." *Human Nature,* April 1978, 60–67.

113. Melzack, Ronald. *The Puzzle of Pain: Revolution in Theory and Treatment.* New York: Basic Books, 1973.

114. Murphy, Marvin L. "Treatment of Chronic Stable Angina: A Preliminary Report of Survival Data of the Randomized Veterans Administration Cooperative Study." *New England Journal of Medicine,* 1977, *297,* 12.

115. Newberne, P. M. "Overnutrition and Resistance of Dogs to Distemper Virus." *Fed. Proc. Fed. Am. Soc. Exp. Biol.,* 1966, *25,* 1701.

116. Old, Lloyd J. "Cancer Immunology." *Scientific American,* May 1977, 62–79

117. Orne, M. T. "The Nature of Hypnosis: Artifact and Essence." *Journal of Abnormal and Social Psychology,* 1959, *58,* 277–99.

118. Ornstein, Robert. *The Psychology of Consciousness.* New York: Harcourt Brace Jovanovich, 1977.

119. Oyle, Irving. *The Healing Mind.* Millbrae, Calif.: Celestial Arts Press, 1975.

120. Parsons, F. M. et al. "Regression of Malignant Tumors in Magnesium and Potassium Depletion Induced by Diet and Hemodialysis." *Lancet,* 1974, *I,* 243–44.

121. Patel, C., and Datey, K. K. "Yoga and Biofeedback in the Management of Hypertension: Two Control Studies." *Proceedings of the Biofeedback Research Society.* Monterey, Calif., 1975.

122. Paton, Bruce C. "Who Needs Coronary Bypass Surgery?" *Human Nature,* September 1978, 76–83.

123. Pauling, Linus. *Vitamin C and the Common Cold.* San Francisco: W. H. Freeman, 1970.

124. Pelletier, Kenneth R. *Mind as Healer, Mind as Slayer: A Holistic Approach to Preventing Stress Disorders.* New York: Delta, 1977.

125. ———, and Garfield, C. *Consciousness East and West.* New York: Harper and Row, 1976.

126. "Personal Safeguards Against Cancer." *Medical Tribune,* November 22, 1978, 1, 6, 22.

127. Pert, A.; Rosenblatt, J. E.; Sivit, C.; Pert, C. B.; and Bunney, W. E., Jr. "Long-term Treatment with Lithium Prevents the

Development of Dopamine Receptor Sensitivity." *Science,* 1978, *201,* 171–73.

128. Peters, R. K.; Benson, H.; and Porter, D. "Daily Relaxation Response Breaks in a Working Population." *American Journal of Public Health,* October 1977, *67,* 946–53.

129. Pomeranz, B., and Chiu, D. "Naloxone Blockade of Acupuncture Analgesia: Endorphin Implicated." *Life Science,* 1976, *19,* 1757–62.

130. Porkert, Manfred. "The Dilemma of Present-day Interpretations of Chinese Medicine." In *Medicine in Chinese Cultures,* ed. A. Kleinman et al. USDHEW, 1975.

131. ———. "The Intellectual and Social Impulses Behind the Evolution of Traditional Chinese Medicine." In *Asian Medical Systems,* Charles Leslie, ed. Berkeley: University of California Press, 1976.

132. ———. "Chinese Medicine: A Traditional Healing Science." In *Ways of Health,* D. S. Sobel, ed. New York: Harcourt Brace Jovanovich, 1979.

133. "Puzzling Pills: Are Placebos Magic or Real?" *Time,* July 30, 1979, 70.

134. Raica, N.; Scott, J.; Lowry, D. S.; and Sauberlich, H. E. "Vitamin A Concentration in Human Tissues Collected from Five Areas in the United States." *American Journal of Clinical Nutrition,* 1972, *25,* 291.

135. Rao, B., and Broadhurst, A. D. "Tryptophan and Depression." *British Medical Journal,* February 21, 1976, *1,* 460.

136. Reichlin, Seymour; Baldessarini, R. J.; and Martin, J. B., eds. *The Hypothalamus.* New York: Raven, 1978. (Research Publications: Association for Research in Nervous and Mental Disease, vol. 56).

137. Relman, A. S. "Holistic Medicine" (editorial). *The New England Journal of Medicine,* February 8, 1979, *300:6,* 312–13.

138. Rhinehart, Luke. *The Book of est.* New York: Holt, Rhinehart, Winston, 1976.

139. Ryle, Gilbert. *The Concept of Mind.* London: Hutchinson, 1949.

140. Sandner, Donald F. "Navaho Medicine." *Human Nature,* July 1978, 54–62.

141. Saward, Ernest, and Sorensen, Andrew. "The Current Emphasis on Preventive Medicine." *Science,* 1978, *200,* 889–94.

142. Scheflen, A. E. "Malignant Tumors in the Institutionalized Psychotic Population." *Arch. Neurol. Psychiat.,* 1951, *64,* 145–55.

143. Schwartz, Gary E. "Biofeedback and the Treatment of Disregulation Disorders." In *Ways of Health,* D. S. Sobel, ed. New York: Harcourt Brace Jovanovich, 1979.

144. Scrimshaw, Nevin S., and Young, Vernon R. "The Requirements of Human Nutrition." *Scientific American,* September 1976, 50–64.

145. Scriver, C. R.; Laberge, C.; Clow, C. L.; and Fraser, F. C.; "Genetics and Medicine: An Evolving Relationship." *Science,* 1978, *200,* 946–52.

146. Selye, Hans. *The Stress of Life.* New York: McGraw-Hill, 1956.

147. ———. Foreword to *Stress and the Art of Biofeedback,* by Barbara B. Brown. New York: Harper and Row, 1977.

148. ———. "They All Looked Sick to Me." *Human Nature,* February 1978, 58–63.

149. Shor, R. E. "Hypnosis and the Concept of the Generalized Reality-Orientation." *American Journal of Psychotherapy,* 1959, *13,* 582–602. Reprinted in *Altered States of Consciousness,* Charles T. Tart, ed. New York: John Wiley and Sons, 1969, pp. 233–50.

150. ———. "Three Dimensions of Hypnotic Depth." *International Journal of Clinical and Experimental Hypnosis,* 1962, *10,* 23–38. Reprinted in *Altered States of Consciousness,* C. T. Tart, ed. New York: John Wiley and Sons, 1969, pp. 251–61.

151. Simonton, O. Carl. "The Role of the Mind in Cancer Therapy." In *The Dimensions of Healing.* Los Altos, Calif.: Academy of Parapsychology and Medicine, 1972.

152. ———, and Simonton S. "Belief Systems and Management of the Emotional Aspects of Malignancy." *Journal of Transpersonal Psychology,* 1975, *7,* 29–47.

153. Simpson, George Gaylord. *The Meaning of Evolution.* New York: Mentor, 1951.

154. Sjolund, B., and Eriksson, M. "Electro-Acupuncture and Endogenous Morphines." *Lancet,* 1976, *I,* 1085.

155. Sklar, L. S., and Anisman, H. "Stress and Coping Factors Influence Tumor Growth." *Science,* 3 August 1979, *205,* 513–15.

156. Snively, W. D., and Thuerbach, J. *Healing Beyond Medicine.* West Nyack, N.Y.: Parker, 1972.

157. Snyder, Paul. *Toward One Science: The Convergence of Traditions.* New York: St. Martin's Press, 1978.

158. Snyder, Solomon H. "Opiate Receptors and Internal Opiates." *Scientific American,* March 1977, 44–56.

159. Sobel, David S., ed. *Ways of Health: Holistic Approaches to Ancient and Contemporary Medicine.* New York: Harcourt Brace Jovanovich, 1979.

160. Solomon. G. F. and Amkraut, A. A. "Emotion, Stress and Immunity." *Frontiers of Radiation Therapy and Oncology,* 1972, 7, 84–86.

161. "Sonic Doom: Can Jet Noise Kill?" *Time,* September 18, 1978.

162. Stein, M.; Schiavi, R. C.; and Camerino, M. "Influence of Brain and Behavior on the Immune System." *Science,* 1976, *191,* 435–40.

163. Sterman, M. B.; Macdonald, L. R.; and Stone, R. "Biofeedback Training of the Sensorimotor EEG Rhythm in Man: Effects on Epilepsy." *Epilepsia,* 1974, *15,* 385–416.

164. ———. "Neurophysiologic and Clinical Studies of Sensorimotor Cortex EEG Feedback Training: Some Effects on Epilepsy." *Seminars in Psychiatry,* 1974, *5,* 507–25.

165. Stone, Irwin. *The Healing Factor: "Vitamin C" Against Disease.* New York: Grosset and Dunlap, 1972.

166. Strawson, P. F. *Individuals: An Essay in Descriptive Metaphysics.* London: Methuen, 1959.

167. Suskind, R. M., ed. *Malnutrition and the Immune Response.* New York: Raven Press, 1977.

168. Tart, Charles T., ed. *Altered States of Consciousness: A Book of Readings.* New York: John Wiley and Sons, 1969.

169. Thomas, C. B. and K. R. Duszynski. "Closeness to Parents and the Family Constellation in a Prospective Study of Five Disease States: Suicide, Mental Illness, Malignant Tumor, Hypertension and Coronary Heart Disease." *The Johns Hopkins Medical Journal,* 1974, *134,* 251–70.

170. Thomas, Lewis. *The Lives of a Cell: Notes of a Biology Watcher.* New York: Viking Press, 1974.

171. ———. *The Medusa and the Snail.* New York: Viking Press, 1979.

172. Tinbergen, N. "Etiology and Stress Disease." *Science,* 1974, *185,* 26.

173. Unschuld, Paul U. "The Social Organization and Ecology of Medical Practice in Taiwan." In *Asian Medical Systems,* ed. Charles Leslie. Berkeley, Calif.: University of California Press, 1976.

174. VanderKamp, H. "A Niochemical Abnormality in Schizophrenia Involving Ascorbic Acid." *International Journal of Neuropsychiatry,* 1960, *2,* 204–6.

175. Volgyesi, F. A. "School for Patients: Hypnosis-therapy and Psycho-prophylaxis." *British Journal of Medical Hypnosis,* 1954, *5,* 8–17.
176. von Feiandt, K., and I. K. Moustgaard. *The Perceptual World.* New York: Academic Press, 1977.
177. Wallace, Robert Keith, and Benson, Herbert. "The Physiology of Meditation." *Scientific American,* February 1972, 84–90.
178. Weiss, J. M.; Glazer, H. I.; Pohorecky, L. A.; Brick, John; and Miller, N. E. "Effects of Chronic Exposure to Stressors on Avoidance-Escape Behavior and on Brain Norepinephrine. *Psychosomatic Medicine,* 1975, *37,* 522–34.
179. Wenger, M. A.; Bagchi, B. K.; and Anand, B. K. "Experiments in India on 'Voluntary' Control of the Heart and Pulse." *Circulation,* 1971, *24,* 1319–27.
180. Wiener, Norbert. *The Human Use of Human Beings.* Boston: Houghton Mifflin, 1954.
181. Williams, Roger J. *Nutrition Against Disease.* New York: Pitman, 1971.
182. ———. "Nutritional Individuality." *Human Nature,* June 1978, 46–63.
183. Winter, J. A. *Why We Get Sick: The Origins of Illness and Anxiety.* New York: Julian Press, 1962.
184. Wixen, Joan D. "Dr. Selye's Stress Theory." *Modern Maturity,* October-November 1978, *21:5,* 10.
185. Worsley, J. R. *Is Acupuncture for You?* New York: Harper and Row, 1973.
186. Yates, John. "Magnesium for a Long (and Social) Life." *Prevention,* March 1979, 77–81.

RECOMMENDED READING

Herbert Benson, *The Relaxation Response*. New York: William Morrow, 1975.

————, *The Mind-Body Effect*. New York: Simon and Schuster, 1979.
Benson teaches Behavioral Medicine at Harvard Medical School and at Beth Israel Hospital in Boston. His early interest in the relaxation response as a means to offset stress was influential on the holistic movement. The more recent book is broader in scope, and includes discussions of non-Western systems of medicine, as well as considerable new work in behavioral medicine and some cogent observations on the matter of patient responsibility.

Barbara B. Brown, *Stress and the Art of Biofeedback*. New York: Bantam, 1978.
A clear explanation of biofeedback techniques and related relaxation techniques.

Emanuel Cheraskin and W. M. Ringsdorf, Jr. (with Arlene Brecher), *Psychodietetics: Food as the Key to Emotional Health*. New York: Bantam, 1976.
A thorough and enthusiastic rundown of recent research which connects diet with emotional states, and an attempt to develop a diet program to promote mental health in particular.

Norman Cousins, *Anatomy of an Illness as Perceived by the Patient*. New York: W. W. Norton, 1979.
Cousins, in his editorials for the *Saturday Review*, has brought holistic approaches to health before the public. In this book, he recounts his personal experience with a serious illness that ultimately responded to a persuasive strategy coupled with large amounts of ascorbic acid. His insights concerning the implications of the holistic health movement are sharp and to the point.

Jerome Frank, *Persuasion and Healing*, rev. ed. Baltimore: Johns Hopkins University Press, 1973.
Frank is Professor Emeritus of Psychiatry at Johns Hopkins. His systematic studies of the role of belief and emotion in healing provide stimulating and informative reading.

Ronald J. Glasser, *The Body Is the Hero*. New York: Random House, 1976.
A clear and thorough explanation of the immune system and the factors which affect it, including some material on emotional influences in the later chapters.

Kenneth R. Pelletier, *Mind as Healer, Mind as Slayer: A Holistic Approach to Preventing Stress Disorders*. New York: Delta, 1977.

————, *Holistic Medicine: From Pathology to Optimum Health*. New York: Delacorte Press/Seymour Lawrence, 1979.
The first book concentrates on stress, the second on the "afflictions of civilization," their prevention and ways to cope with them. Clear, cogent, and useful books.

Ralph Ruddock, ed., *Six Approaches to the Person*. London: Routledge & Kegan Paul, 1972.
>   Although there is nothing here of direct medical relevance, these six essays will be of interest to those who want to explore the philosophical concept of a *person*.

David S. Sobel, ed., *Ways of Health: Holistic Approaches to Ancient and Contemporary Medicine*. New York: Harcourt Brace Jovanovich, 1979.
>   A serious and varied collection of articles by established medical researchers on all the major topics of holistic health. Highly recommended.

Lewis Thomas, *Lives of a Cell: Notes of a Biology Watcher*. New York: Viking Press, 1974.

————, *The Medusa and the Snail*. New York: Viking Press, 1979.
>   Both of these books are primarily collections of Thomas' columns from the *New England Journal of Medicine*. Thomas is President of Memorial Sloan-Kettering Cancer Center in New York City. While he is not directly caught up in the holistic movement, his thoroughly sensible, informative, and insightful essays give a good perspective on contemporary medical thought. Thomas cautions against some of the simplistic approaches to health care that have arisen recently, and cautions against letting a good idea run away with itself. In addition, these are some of the best-written essays on any subject to appear in a long time.

Roger J. Williams. *Nutrition Against Disease*. New York: Pitman, 1971.
>   Williams emphasizes individual differences in nutritional needs, and takes a sensible, careful approach to estimating dietary needs.

HOLISTIC HEALTH ORGANIZATIONS

The following organizations are included in a list compiled and published by the *Holistic Health Review* and are possible sources of information. Reprinted with permission; copyright © 1980, *Holistic Health Review*, 1030 Merced St., Berkeley, CA 94707.

Alternative Medical Association, 7916 S.E. Stark, Portland, OR 97215

American Holistic Medical Association, Route 2, Welsh Coulee, La Crosse, WI 54601

Association for Humanistic Gerontology, 1711 Solano Ave, Berkeley, CA 94707

Association for Humanistic Psychology, 325 Ninth Street, San Francisco, CA 94103

Austin Area Holistic Health Association, P.O. Box 13281, Austin, TX 78711

The Canadian Holistic Healing Association, 308 E. 23rd Ave, Vancouver, B.C., Canada

Cancer Control Society, 2043 North Berendo, Los Angeles, CA 90027

Cancer Counseling and Research Center, Suite 720, 1300 Summit Ave, Fort Worth, TX 76102

Center for Integral Medicine, 1515 Palisades Dr, Pacific Palisades, CA 90272

Center for Science in the Public Interest, 1755 S Street, N.W., Washington, D.C. 20009

Citizens' Energy Project, 1110 Sixth Street, N.W., Washington, D.C. 20001

Committee for Integrated Health, P.O. Box 483, Davis, CA 95616

Colorado Holistic Health Network, Suite 526, Mercy Hospital, East 16th and Milwaukee Streets, Denver, CO 80218

Eastern Area Association for Holistic Health, 50 Maple Pl., Manhasset, NY 11030

Holistic Health Association of the Princeton Area, 360 Nassau, Princeton, NJ 08540

Holistic Health Practitioners' Association, 1030 Merced Street, Berkeley, CA 94707

Human Dimensions in Medical Education, 1125 Torrey Pines Road, La Jolla, CA 92037

Institute for Holistic Health and Education, 1220 Sansom Street, Philadelphia, PA 19107

The Institute for the Study of Human Knowledge, P.O. Box 176, Los Altos, CA 94011

International Federation on Ageing, 1909 K Street, N.W., Washington, D.C. 20049

National Health Federation, P.O. Box 688, Monrovia, CA 91016

Nurses in Transition, P.O. Box 14472, San Francisco, CA 94114

Orenda Association for Holistic Health, 1742 N. Opdyke, Auburn Heights, MI 48057

Sacramento Holistic Health Association, 1616 21st Street, Sacramento, CA 95814

Tucson Holistic Health Association, 300 E. River Road, Tucson, AZ 85704

Unity-in-Diversity Council, 7433 Madora Avenue, Canoga Park, CA 91306

Vegetarian Association of America, P.O. Box 86, Livingston, NJ 07039

Washington Association for Holistic Health, P.O. Box 7123, Olympia, WA 98507

SUBJECT INDEX

Acetylcholine, 96
Activity
  habits of, 219, 276–292
  vs. process, 14
Acupuncture, 105, 108–117
  in animals, 112, 114
  Eastern medicine and, 105, 108,
    114–115
  effectiveness of, 114, 115
  meridians and points in, 109–110,
    116
  neurochemicals and, 116–117
  pain and, 115–117
  placebo effect in, 114
  stress and, 117
  Western discovery of, 113–115
Adaptation, 20–21, 25–32, 65–69,
    84–85, 123–124
  of individual, 25–26, 30, 65–69,
    84–85, 123–124
  of medical system, 117, 119–120
  stress and, 25–29
Aflatoxin, 187
African healing traditions, 82, 106
Airport noise and stress, 138–139
Alpha state, 52, 54, 144, 147, 148, 151
Altered states of consciousness,
    101–102, 149, 206–207. *See also*
    Meditation; Hypnosis
American Indians, 105–106
Ames test, 134
Amphetamines, 93–94
"Anniversary syndrome," 66–67
Antigens, 35
"Appropriate Technology," 217–218
Arthritis, 26, 29, 84, 203
Ascorbic acid, 125, 174–180, 184
  as antiseptic, 178
  in colds, 174–175
  in collagen production, 176
  immune system and, 177–178
  metabolism and, 176
  need, estimates, 179–180
  nervous system and, 176–177
  smoking and, 177
  stress and, 175–176

Ascorbic acid *(continued)*
  synthesis of, 175, 179
Attitude and health, 16, 53–57,
    220–221
Auto-immune disease, 24
Autonomic nervous system, 142, 152

Bacterial tests, 134
Balance studies (nutrients), 168
Barefoot doctors, 119–120
Beef, 130–132, 189–190
  and intestinal cancer, 130–132
Behaviorism, 11–12, 203–204
Belief, 54–55, 82–83, 107
Biochemical habits, 98–100
Biofeedback, 141–146, 211–213
  animals and, 143
  in blood pressure control, 143
  clinical uses of, 145–146
  epilepsy and, 144
  meditation and, 145–146
  paralysis and, 144
  stress and, 144
Biological heritage, 19–32, 46–47,
    84–85, 152, 165–167, 178–179,
    199, 208–209, 215
Biological responses, 22–29, 83–86,
    88–89, 101–102, 103–104. *See*
    also Immune response; Fight-or-
    flight response; Relaxation response
"Blaming the victim," 67–69
Blood pressure, 26, 28, 143, 148, 150,
    155, 211–213, 219
  biofeedback and, 143, 147
  other diseases and, 154
  prevention, 154–155
  relaxation response and, 150–155,
    211–212
  treatment, 153–154, 211–212
Brain, 87–102, 183. *See also*
    Neurochemistry
  as chemical system, 88–98
  as computer, 91–92
  function, 88–98, 101, 183
Breathing, control of, 141–142

238

NAME INDEX